# The Labor Progress Handbook

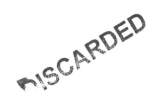

# The Labor Progress Handbook
## Early Interventions to Prevent and Treat Dystocia

**Penny Simkin**   *BA, PT, CCE, CD (DONA)*
*Seattle Midwifery School*
*Independent Practice of Childbirth Education and*
*Labor Support*

**Ruth Ancheta**   *BA, ICCE, CD (DONA)*
*Independent Practice of Childbirth Education and*
*Labor Support*

with

**Jilly Rosser**   *MEd, RM*
*Midwifery Consultant*

*Illustrated by* **Shanna Dela Cruz**

Blackwell
Science

618.5
Sim

© 2000 by
Blackwell Science Ltd

Copyright for illustrations 1994 and
    1999 Ruth Ancheta

Blackwell Science Ltd
Osney Mead, Oxford OX2 0EL

The right of the Authors to be identified as
the Authors of this Work has been asserted
in accordance with the Copyright, Designs
and Patents Act 1988.

A catalogue record for this title
is available from the British Library

ISBN 0-632-05281-3

Library of Congress
Cataloging-in-Publication Data
Simkin, Penny, 1938–
    The labor progress handbook: early
    interventions to prevent and treat
    dystocia/Penny Simkin, Ruth Ancheta,
    with Jilly Rosser.
        p.    cm.
    Includes bibliographical references
and index.
    ISBN 0-632-05281-3 (pbk.)
    1. Birth injuries – Prevention
Handbooks, manuals, etc.   2. Labor
(Obstetrics) – Complications
Handbooks, manuals, etc.
3. Pregnancy – Complications
Handbooks, manuals, etc.   I. Ancheta,
Ruth.   II. Rosser, Jilly.   III. Title.
RG701.S57   1999
618.5 – dc21                    99-25452
                                      CIP

DISTRIBUTORS

Marston Book Services Ltd
PO Box 269
Abingdon
Oxon OX14 4YN
(Orders: Tel: 01235 465500
            Fax: 01235 465555)

USA
Blackwell Science, Inc.
Commerce Place
350 Main Street
Malden, MA 02148 5018
(Orders: Tel: 800 759 6102
            781 388 8250
    Fax: 781 388 8255)

Canada
Login Brothers Book Company
324 Saulteaux Crescent
Winnipeg, Manitoba R3J 3T2
(Orders: Tel: 204 837 2987
            Fax: 204 837 3116)

Australia
Blackwell Science Pty Ltd
54 University Street
Carlton, Victoria 3053
(Orders: Tel: 03 9347 0300
            Fax: 03 9347 5001)

For further information on Blackwell
Science, visit our website:
www.blackwell-science.com

First published 2000
Reprinted 2000, 2001

Set in 9/11 pt Plantin
by DP Photosetting, Aylesbury, Bucks
Printed and bound in the UK by
MPG Books Ltd, Bodmin, Cornwall

**Please note**

The information in this book was compiled from published research findings and clinical experience of doctors, midwives, nurses, doulas, anthropologists, childbirth educators, the authors, and others. The approach to dysfunctional labor and the solutions suggested here should be considered in the context of each specific case. Since nothing in this book is intended as medical advice, clinical care providers should assess the suggestions for their applicability to the particular situation.

# Contents

# Foreword

At last, a book that offers practical advice for nurses and midwives who wish to help to prevent and treat dysfunctional labor! Penny Simkin and Ruth Ancheta have done a superb job of interweaving the clinical wisdom of observant, expert practitioners with the best available research evidence about what helps and does not help women during labor.

I wish this book had been available a long time ago. In the early 1970s when I was a novice labor and delivery nurse, I observed a common but puzzling problem. In those days we subjected women to an admission routine that included a variety of very unpleasant procedures. (Thankfully the worst of these procedures – perineal shaves, enemas, and rectal exams – have since been recognized as useless or harmful and have been eliminated from common practice.) Part of the admission routine involved assessment of the quality and strength of contractions. When I inquired about the contractions, I was often told, 'My contractions were frequent and strong at home, but they seem to have gotten a lot weaker and further apart since I arrived.'

I would reply, 'Do not worry, this happens a lot. After we finish the admission procedures and you are settled in here, your labor will probably get going again.'

Why did I say this? I believed it. I had observed it often and had overheard experienced colleagues reassure their patients in this way. At some intuitive level I felt the decrease in labor intensity was caused by the woman's reaction to the stress of the hospital admission routine. But at the time almost nothing had been written about the role of stress hormones on uterine function, nor about the relationships between maternal anxiety, environmental influences, stress hormones, and labor complications. And the randomized controlled trials showing the substantial benefits of labor support had not even been conducted yet[1].

What about the instances in which labor did not return

spontaneously to the strong, regular pattern that had been occurring prior to admission? Our repertoire of nursing interventions was limited primarily to advising the woman either to ambulate or to rest and wait. (Currently in some settings the options may be even fewer, with ambulation restricted by the routine use of electronic fetal monitors.) These women frequently ended up with a cascade of medical interventions – I-V oxytocin, amniotomy, epidural analgesia, and forceps or cesarean delivery.

I now believe that there is much more I could have done to prevent or treat the problem of dysfunctional labor. Penny Simkin and Ruth Ancheta have described how 'emotional dystocia' and stressful environmental influences may lead to complications, and they offer simple but potentially powerful nursing measures to ameliorate these problems. They have also persuaded me that many instances of dystocia or prolonged labor may be caused by subtle malpositions of the fetal head, potentially correctable with simple positioning techniques.

I can only imagine how much more effective I would have been if this book had been available when I was a labor and delivery nurse. As a researcher, I am inspired to study these simple but potentially very powerful labor support techniques. Dystocia or dysfunctional labor is the most common reason for primary cesarean delivery. Given the high rates of cesarean delivery in North America and the UK, and the limitations and risks of medical treatments for dystocia, it seems long overdue that nurses and midwives take an active role in preventing and treating this common clinical problem. This book contains a wealth of information about and practical suggestions for preventing and correcting dysfunctional labor. It should be required reading for all who care for women in labor, and a reference text in every labor and birthing unit.

Ellen D. Hodnett *RN, PhD*
*Professor and Heather M. Reisman Chair*
*Perinatal Nursing Research*
*University of Toronto*

## REFERENCE

1. Hodnett E. Support from caregivers during childbirth (Cochrane Review). In: *The Cochrane Library*, Issue 3, 1998. Update Software, Oxford.

We dedicate this book to childbearing women and their caregivers in the hope that some of our suggestions will reduce the likelihood of cesarean delivery for dystocia.

## Acknowledgements

We have been helped in writing this book by many wonderful people, especially:

- Sally Avenson, Roberta Gehrke, Lynn Diulio, Mary Mazul, Jean Sutton, Karen Hillegas, Barbara Kalmen, Karen Kohls, Ann Krigbaum, Karen Lupa, and Suzy Myers for their helpful suggestions;
- John Carroll, Alicia Huntley, Shauna Leinbach, Jenny McAllister, and Sara Wickham for reviewing the text and giving us useful feedback;
- Diony Young, for her assistance and support;
- Shanna dela Cruz, our dedicated and meticulous illustrator;
- the dozens of women and men who posed for our illustrations, especially Robin Block, Asela Calhoun, Vic dela Cruz, Helen Vella Dentice, Maureen Wahhab, Bob Meidl and Lori Meidl Zahorodney, and staff members of Waukesha Memorial Hospital and St. Mary's Hospital of Milwaukee, Wisconsin, USA;
- Lesley James, Jan Dowers and Tracy Sachtjen, who provided support and assistance with word processing, communication, and other ways of making our lives easier;
- last but not least, our families who have helped us in countless ways as we devoted ourselves to this larger than expected task.

# Chapter 1
# **Introduction**

Labor dystocia, dysfunctional labor, failure to progress – all these terms refer to slow or no progress in labor, which is one of the most vexing, complex and unpredictable complications of labor. Labor dystocia is the most common indication for primary cesarean sections, and in countries where rates of vaginal births after previous cesareans are relatively low (for example, in the United States in 1996 this figure was less than 30%[1]), dystocia also contributes indirectly to the number of repeat cesareans. It is clear that prevention of dystocia would not only reduce the number of costly and risky obstetric interventions, including cesareans, but it would also spare some women from the feelings of discouragement and disappointment that often accompany a prolonged or complicated birth.

The possible causes of labor dystocia are numerous. Some are intrinsic:

- The *powers* (the uterine contractions)
- The *passage* (size, shape, and joint mobility of the pelvis and the stretch and resilience of the vaginal canal)
- The *passenger* (size and shape of fetal head, fetal presentation and position)
- The *pain* (and the woman's ability to cope with it)
- The *psyche* (anxiety, emotional state of the woman).

**1**

Others are extrinsic:

- *Environment* (the feelings of physical and emotional safety generated by the setting and the people surrounding the woman)
- *Ethno-cultural factors* (the degree of sensitivity and respect for the woman's culture-based needs and preferences)
- *Hospital or caregiver policies* (how flexible, family- or woman-centered, evidence based)
- *Psycho-emotional care* (the priority given to non-clinical aspects of the childbirth experience).

*The Labor Progress Handbook* focuses on prevention, differential diagnosis, and early interventions to use in dysfunctional labor. The emphasis is on relatively simple and sensible care measures or interventions designed to help maintain normal labor progress and to manage and correct minor complications before they become serious enough to require major interventions.

The suggestions in this book are based on the following premises:

- Progress may slow or stop for any of a number of reasons at any time in labor – pre-labor, early labor, active labor, or during the second or third stage.
- The timing of the delay is an important consideration when establishing cause and selecting interventions.
- Sometimes several causal factors may occur at one time.
- Caregivers and others are often able to enhance or maintain labor progress with simple non-surgical, non-pharmacological physical and psychological interventions. Such interventions have the following advantages:
  - ○ compared to most obstetric interventions for dystocia, they carry less risk of harm or undesirable side effects to mother or baby
  - ○ they treat the woman as the key to the solution, not the key to the problem
  - ○ they build or strengthen the cooperation between the woman, her support people (loved ones, doula), and caregivers
  - ○ they reduce the need for riskier, costlier, more complex interventions
  - ○ they may increase the woman's emotional satisfaction with her experience of birth.

- The choice of solutions depends on the causal factors, if known, but trial and error is sometimes necessary when the cause is unclear. The greatest drawbacks are that the woman may not want to try these interventions, they sometimes take time, or they may not correct the problem.
- Time is usually an ally, not an enemy. With time, many problems in labor progress are resolved. In the absence of clear medical or psychological contraindications, patience, reassurance and low or no risk interventions may constitute the most appropriate course of management.
- The caregiver may use the following in determining the cause of the problem(s):
    - *objective observations:* woman's vital signs; fetal heart rate patterns; fetal presentation, position and size; cervical assessments; assessments of contraction strength, frequency, and duration; membrane status; and time
    - *subjective observations:* woman's affect, description of pain, level of fatigue
    - *direct questions* of the woman and *collaboration* with her in decisions regarding treatment:

        'What was going through your mind during that contraction?'
        'Please describe your pain.'
        'Why do you think labor has slowed down?'
        'Which options for treatment do you prefer?'

- Once the probable cause and the woman's perceptions and views are determined, appropriate primary interventions are instituted and labor progress is further observed. The problem may be solved with no further interventions.
- If the primary interventions are medically contraindicated or if they are unsuccessful, then obstetrical interventions are instituted under the guidance of the doctor or midwife.

Chart 1.1 illustrates the approach described in this book. Other similar flow charts appear throughout this book to illustrate the application of this approach to a variety of causes of dysfunctional labor.

Many of the interventions described in this book are derived from the medical, midwifery, nursing, and childbirth education literature. Others come from the psychology, sociology, and anthropology liter-

**1**

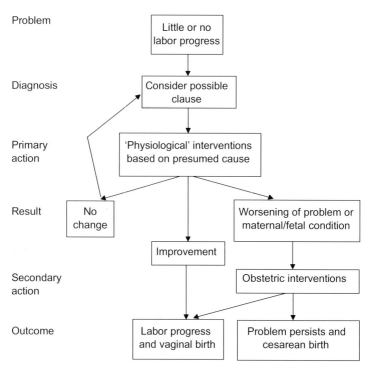

| | |
|---|---|
| Problem | Little or no labor progress |
| Diagnosis | Consider possible clause |
| Primary action | 'Physiological' interventions based on presumed cause |
| Result | No change / Worsening of problem or maternal/fetal condition |
| | Improvement |
| Secondary action | Obstetric interventions |
| Outcome | Labor progress and vaginal birth / Problem persists and cesarean birth |

**Chart 1.1**   Care Plan for the Problem, 'Little or No Labor Progress'.

ature. We have provided references for these, when available. Some suggestions have come from the extensive experience of nurses, midwives, doctors, and doulas (labor support providers). Many are applications of physical therapy principles and practices. Some items fall into the category of 'shared wisdom', where the original sources are unknown. We apologize if we neglect to mention the originator of an idea that has become widespread enough to fall into this category. Finally, some ideas originated with one or both of the authors who have used them successfully in their work with laboring women.

With today's emphasis on evidence-based practice, many rather entrenched maternity care customs are falling out of favor because they have been proven ineffective or harmful. Such routine practices as enemas, pubic shaving, continuous electronic fetal monitoring without access to fetal scalp blood sampling, the use of maternal supine and lithotomy positions in the second stage of labor, and routine episiotomy are some examples of forms of care that became widespread before they were scientifically evaluated. Then, once well-controlled trials of safety and effectiveness had been performed and the results combined in meta-analyses, these common practices were found to be ineffective and to increase risks.[2]

Where possible, we will base our suggestions on such scientific evidence and will cite appropriate references. However, numerous simple and apparently risk-free practices have never been scientifically studied. Some of these are based on an understanding of the emotional and physiological processes taking place during childbirth. Others are applications of anatomy, kinesiology, and body mechanics to enhance the relationships between such separate but interdependent forces as pelvic shape, maternal posture, fetal position and station, uterine activity, and the force of gravity. Still others are based on a recognition of the importance of each laboring woman's personal and cultural values.

Some of the strategies suggested in this book will lend themselves well to randomized controlled trials, while others may not. Perhaps readers will gather ideas for scientific study as they read this book and apply its suggestions.

## SOME IMPORTANT DIFFERENCES IN MATERNITY CARE BETWEEN THE UNITED STATES, THE UNITED KINGDOM, AND CANADA

This book is being published simultaneously in North America and the United Kingdom, where the approaches to maternity care are quite different from one another. It may surprise the reader to read about some of those differences, and it may also be interesting to learn that practices that are considered essential for safety in one country are considered ineffective or archaic in another. We hope that one side effect of our book will be to encourage a willingness to reconsider practices that are either entrenched or avoided in one's own workplace.

Table 1.1 compares some basic features of maternity care between the United States, Canada, and the United Kingdom.

With such differences in maternity care as those listed in Table 1.1, the willingness to introduce new practices and the power to do so will

**Table 1.1**  Comparison of maternity care in the United States, Canada, and the United Kingdom.

| Feature | United States | Canada | United Kingdom |
|---------|---------------|--------|----------------|
| Primary maternity caregivers | Obstetricians for approximately 90% of women; midwives and family physicians for 10%. Maternity nurses provide most of the care during labor in the hospital, with the obstetrician managing any problems and the delivery. | Family physicians, with obstetricians and recently legalized midwives now increasing in numbers. As in the USA, nurses provide most in-hospital care. | Mostly midwives, some general practitioners, with obstetricians caring for women with complications. There are no maternity nurses. Midwives provide all intrapartum care and conduct most deliveries. |
| Autonomy and independence of caregiver | Great variation in preferred routines among independent physicians. Nursing care varies according to the orders of each physician. Insurance providers and health maintenance organizations now increasingly limit those physicians' practices that are not cost-effective. | Government limits payment for some interventions, and regulates numbers of doctors and hospitals, giving doctors less autonomy than in the USA. | Midwives have little autonomy, and practice according to the policies of their institutions. Those policies are established by authorities in maternity care and by the government. |
| Participation by childbearing women in decision-making | 'Informed consent' is the law, though most women (except assertive women with strong opinions) expect the obstetrician to make decisions and most obstetricians prefer that style of practice. Most midwives and family physicians share decision-making with the woman. | Similar to the USA. | 'Informed choice' and 'woman-centered care' are now standards of care, and extensive efforts are being made by government and childbirth activists to ensure that women are well informed for their role as partners in decision-making. |

*Contd*

**Table 1.1** *Contd*

| | | | |
|---|---|---|---|
| Continuity of caregiver throughout the childbearing year | Not considered cost-effective, feasible, or desirable by policy-makers in health care. Rarely available except for out of hospital births, though to many women it is a highly desirable option. Some assertive women try to obtain continuity of care through birth plans and doulas, and by verbalizing their concerns to each professional involved in their care. | Small group practices of family physicians are available in many parts of Canada. Continuity of caregiver during pregnancy and post partum is more likely than in the USA, although maternity nurses provide most care in labor. | Considered a very important feature of woman-centered care, programs ensuring continuity of caregiver are beginning to replace the old system of different midwives for pre- and postnatal and intrapartum care. |
| Influence of scientific evidence on maternity practices | Highly variable, but customs, opinions and prior experience of the practitioner and fear of litigation are more powerful influences. Some medical, nursing, and midwifery schools now teach and follow principles of evidence-based practice. | Leaders in obstetrics, family medicine, and nursing are actively engaged in scientific evaluation of numerous unproved clinical practices. The Society of Obstetricians and Gynecologists of Canada promotes evidence-based practice. | Same as Canada, except that midwives are also actively involved in research. There is widespread acceptance of a scientific approach to maternity care, where possible. |
| Influence of fear of malpractice litigation on maternity practices | The likelihood of doctors being sued for malpractice is high, and malpractice insurance premiums are extremely expensive, which has driven up the costs of maternity care. In addition, insurers advise on how to reduce the likelihood of lawsuits. Such advice (e.g. to use continuous electronic fetal monitoring, and perform cesareans frequently) is not based on science, safety or effectiveness, but on risks of being sued. | Trends similar to the USA, although to a much lesser degree. Fear of litigation has less impact on care than scientific findings, costs, customs and other factors. | Similar to Canada. |

**1**

vary among caregivers in different countries. We hope our readers will begin to utilize the simplest, most innocuous measures immediately, and to educate themselves and change policies where necessary, so that the other more complex or expensive techniques can also be evaluated and utilized.

## NOTES ON THIS BOOK

This book is directed toward midwives, nurses, and doctors who want to support and enhance the physiological process of labor with the objective of avoiding complex, costly, more risky interventions. It will also be helpful for students in obstetrics, midwifery, and maternity nursing, for childbirth educators who can teach many of these techniques to expectant parents, and for doulas (trained labor support providers). The chapters are arranged chronologically according to the phases and stages of labor.

Because a particular maternal position or movement is useful for the same problem during more than one phase of labor, we have included illustrations of these positions in more than one chapter. This will allow the reader to find position ideas at a glance when working with a laboring woman. Complete descriptions of all the positions, movements, and other measures can be found in the 'Toolkit', Chapters 6 and 7.

The term 'caregiver' is used to refer to any of the people mentioned above who are providing care and support for the woman in labor.

## CONCLUSION

The current emphasis in obstetrics is to find better ways to treat dystocia once it occurs. Little emphasis is placed on prevention, which is the focus of this book.

To our knowledge, this is the first book that compiles labor progress strategies that can be used by a variety of caregivers in a variety of locations. Most of the strategies described can be used for births occurring in hospitals, at home, and in out-of-hospital birth centers.

It is hoped that this book will make your work more effective and more rewarding. Your knowledge of appropriate early interventions may spare many women from long, discouraging, or exhausting labors, reduce the need for major interventions, and contribute to safer and more satisfying outcomes. The women may not even recognize what you have done for them, but they will appreciate and always remember your attentiveness, expertise, and support, which contribute so much to positive long-term memories of their childbirths[3].

We wish you much success and fulfillment in your important work.

## REFERENCES

1. Center for Disease Control/National Center for Health Statistics (1998) *Monthly Vital Statistics Report, 1995–1998.* CDC, Atlanta.
2. Enkin, M. Keirse, M.J.N.C., Renfrew, M. & Neilson, J. (1995) *A Guide to Effective Care in Pregnancy and Childbirth*, 2nd edn. Oxford University Press, Oxford.
3. Simkin, P. (1990) Just another day in a woman's life? Women's long term perceptions of their first birth experience. Part I. *Birth* **18(4)**, 203–10.

# Chapter 2
# Dysfunctional Labor: General Considerations

**2**

## WHAT IS DYSFUNCTIONAL LABOR?

The term 'dysfunctional labor' is a catch-all term that refers to protracted or arrested progress in cervical dilation in the active phase of labor, or protracted or arrested descent in the second stage. Other terms, such as 'labor dystocia', 'uterine inertia' 'persistent malposition', 'cephalo-pelvic disproportion', 'failure to progress', and 'protracted labor', or as some clinicians have said in frustration, 'WCO' ('won't come out!'), have been used to refer to dysfunctional labor. Some caregivers are less patient than others and diagnose dystocia more quickly.

Diagnosis and management of dysfunctional labor vary, depending on the philosophy of the care provider. For example, proponents of 'active management of labor' begin high dose oxytocin augmentation of nulliparas any time after labor is diagnosed, if the rate of dilation is less than 1 cm/hour for 2 hours[1]. Other caregivers diagnose dysfunctional labor only after the active phase has commenced and the rate of dilation is less than 0.5 cm/hour for 4 hours[2]. Others individualize their approach to dystocia and base their actions on a variety of clinical and non-clinical factors. If the woman can be made comfortable and the fetus shows few or no signs of distress, they feel less urgency to speed progress. They may consider other factors in deciding when, whether, and how to intervene, for example, the cause of the slow progress and the likelihood that the problem will resolve itself by waiting, the adequacy of staffing now and later, their own availability, and the woman's needs or desires. Still others, including many midwives, try very hard to avoid augmentation with oxytocin by ensuring the privacy of the woman by nourishing, supporting and reassuring her, and by exercising patience and watchful waiting to allow the labor process to unfold at its own pace.

## MAINTAINING LABOR PROGRESS: PREVENTION OF DYSFUNCTIONAL LABOR

The first principle in management of labor dystocia is prevention. By keeping in mind the *psycho-emotional*, *physical*, and *physiological* factors that are important in maintaining good labor progress, the caregiver can often prevent dystocia.

## THE PSYCHO-EMOTIONAL STATE OF THE WOMAN: REDUCING MATERNAL DISTRESS

Labor progress is facilitated when a woman feels safe, respected, and cared for by the experts who are responsible for her clinical safety, and when her pain is adequately and safely managed. Her partner or loved ones and her caregivers contribute significantly to such feelings. The opposite – feelings of shame or embarrassment, of being observed, of being in danger, being treated with disrespect, feeling ignored or insignificant – may elicit a psychobiological reaction that interferes with efficient progress in labor.

Michel Odent, MD, an observer and student of normal birth since the early 1960s, has postulated that when women give birth 'in the method of the mammals' their labors are more likely to proceed without difficulty. Because birth involves primitive parts of the brain that humans share with other mammals, he advocates modifying present-day facilities and care practices to allow women to turn off the newer and more uniquely human part of the brain, the neocortex. He notes that other mammals seek privacy, a comfortable, cozy, quiet space, and dim light when they are about to give birth. Such an environment reduces activity in the neocortex and allows the mid-brain and brain stem to set in motion the processes mediated by prostaglandins and hormones that enhance the birthing process. Odent points out that today's maternity facilities constantly stimulate the neocortex (bright lights, strangers, many questions, unfamiliar sights and sounds, and more) and inhibit the functioning of the primitive parts of the brain, thus contributing to dystocia[3].

The well-known 'fight or flight' response, a physiological process that promotes survival of the endangered or frightened animal or human, is initiated by the outpouring of catecholamines or stress hormones, such as epinephrine (adrenalin), norepinephrine (noradrenalin), cortisol, and others. Triggered by physical danger, fear, anxiety, or other forms of distress, the fight or flight response has the potential of slowing labor progress (Fig. 2.1). During most of the first stage of labor, excessively high levels of circulating catecholamines cause maternal blood to be shunted away from the uterus and placenta and other organs not essential for immediate survival, to the heart, lungs, brain, and skeletal muscle, the organs essential to fight or flight. The decreased blood supply to the uterus and placenta slows uterine contractions[4] and decreases the availability of oxygen to the fetus[5]. Fear or anxiety also causes the woman to interpret caregivers' words or labor events in a pessimistic or negative way. Avoidance or reduction of maternal psychological distress or enhancement of the woman's sense of well-being appears to facilitate the physiological labor process. Interestingly, an outpouring of catecholamines in late first stage or close to birth has the opposite effect of speeding the birth by causing the 'fetal ejection reflex'[6]. In fact, many women briefly exhibit fear, anger, or even euphoria, typical catecholamine responses, just before the birth[3].

Following are measures a caregiver may use to enhance the woman's

**Maternal effects of anxiety ('fight or flight' response) in labor**

Excessive catecholamine levels in first stage labor cause:

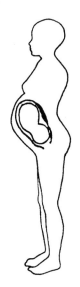

- ↓ blood flow to uterus
- ↓ uterine contractions
- ↑ duration of first stage labor
- ↓ blood flow to placenta
- ↓ oxygen available to fetus
- ↑ fetal production of catecholamines
  - fetal conservation of oxygen
  - fetal heart rate decelerations
- ↑ negative or pessimistic perception of events by woman

Excessive catecholamine levels in second stage labor causes:

- same fetal effects as listed above
- 'fetal ejection reflex' (rapid expulsion of fetus)

**Fig. 2.1** Potential effects of maternal distress.

feelings of security and reduce the likelihood of a detrimental fight or flight response.

## Psycho-emotional measures

*Before labor*

- Before birth, in childbirth classes and in conversations with her midwife or doctor, encourage each woman to think about personally comforting things she and her partner might do or have available in labor, for example, favorite music, scents, or pictures, loved ones or a doula, her own clothing to wear during labor, plans to use visualizations or massage or relaxation techniques. All these may contribute to her sense of familiarity and comfort in her environment. Of course, most of these are easily available in a home birth, but will require some advanced planning and packing for a hospital birth. Some parents write a letter or 'birth plan' to the staff, introducing themselves and describing some of their preferences and choices regarding their care.

- If, as in the USA and Canada (and some areas of the UK), the woman is not acquainted with the nurse and midwife or doctor, check her chart for psychosocial history as well as her clinical situation.

*During labor*

- Introduce yourself by name, and call her by name. Greet and orient her and her support team as appropriate to her needs and stage of labor. Introduce her to the unit (room, lighting, use of bed, bath or shower, call buttons, kitchen, nurses' station, lounge). Try to convey a sense of hospitality and friendliness, along with safety and competence.

- Ask about her plans and preferences. Try to be supportive of her wishes. Does she have a birth plan or preference list? If her wishes are somewhat unrealistic, discuss them kindly and respectfully, offering the choices you can provide.

- Encourage an atmosphere of privacy, comfort, and intimacy between her and her support people:
  ○ knock before entering and keep door closed
  ○ do not leave her body exposed
  ○ tell her what comfort devices you have available (ice pack, hot pack, warm blankets, birth ball, beanbag chair, bath, shower, juices, tea, music tapes, others)
  ○ encourage cuddling, hugging, 'slow dancing'
  ○ encourage and reassure the woman and try to remain with her as much as she wishes and as much as your other responsibilities allow

- Explain any clinical procedures or tests. Give her the results. If the woman's vital signs, her labor progress, and the fetus appear normal, reassure her by telling her so.

- Inform her of the signs of progress as you identify them. See page 31 for information on the six ways to progress.

- Suggest comfort measures to help her cope with labor.

- Reassure her, not only with words, but also, as culturally appropriate, with praise, smiles, touch, hand-holding, or gestures of kindness and respect. These psycho-emotional measures create an atmosphere in which the woman feels well-cared for and they have the added advantages of taking little time and costing next to nothing.

## Physical comfort measures

Using simple physical comfort measures may increase the woman's sense of mastery and reduce her stress and the likelihood of a labor-slowing fight or flight response.

- Create an atmosphere that encourages the woman's spontaneous self-comforting behaviors and those learned in childbirth class:
  - relaxation techniques/rhythmic movements
  - calming vocalizations (moans, sighs)
  - breathing techniques (see Chapter 7, page 195)
  - guided imagery/visualization

- Give her partner suggestions to use as long as they are acceptable to the woman:
  - massage
  - timing contractions or counting her breaths through each one to encourage rhythm and help her know where she is in the contraction (middle or end)
  - wiping her face and neck with a cool cloth
  - words of praise, encouragement
  - speaking in a low rhythmic tone of voice

- Encourage the woman or couple to use available amenities, such as:
  - hot or cold packs
  - bath or shower
  - birth ball

- ○ ice machine, beverages
- ○ lounge
- ○ tape or compact disc player, television

## Physiological measures

The following basic physiological measures also tend to prevent underlying factors that can lead to dystocia.

- Encourage her to empty her bladder hourly. A distended bladder may increase pain or interfere with descent. Contractions sometimes reduce one's awareness of a full bladder, so she may need to be reminded.

- Make sure the woman remains well hydrated, but not over-hydrated. While most laboring women do not need intravenous (I-V) fluids for adequate hydration and prevention of aspiration of gastric contents[7,8], it is policy in many North American and British hospitals to place some restrictions on oral food and fluids, even in healthy uncomplicated pregnancies, and to give I-V fluids instead[9]. Until those policies are changed, be sure that you do not cause overhydration with a too rapid infusion of fluids. Have a variety of juices, frozen juice bars, teas, and water available for oral hydration.

- Encourage the woman to seek comfort, that is, to try a variety of movements and positions and use those in which she feels less pain. The most comfortable movements and positions seem to be ones that also enhance labor progress[10].

- Encourage the woman to relax her voluntary muscles, particularly those in her buttocks, pelvic floor, thighs, abdomen, and low back.

## WHY FOCUS ON MATERNAL POSITION?

In late pregnancy, changes in hormone production relax the ligaments and cartilage of the pelvic joints, allowing greater mobility in the sacro-iliac joints and the pubic symphysis[11]. Pelvic mobility allows for subtle changes in the shape and size of the pelvis, which may facilitate an optimal position of the fetal head in the first stage, as well as the cardinal movements of flexion, internal rotation, and fetal descent in the second stage.

Changes in the woman's position may have beneficial effects on the following:

(1) Alignment of pelvic bones and resulting shape and capacity of the pelvis[11].
(2) Frequency, length, and efficiency of contractions[10].
(3) 'Drive angle' (Figs 2.2a, b), that is, the angle formed by the axis of the fetus' spine and the axis of the birth canal[12].
(4) Effects of gravity[10].
(5) Oxygen supply to fetus[10].

**2**

(a)

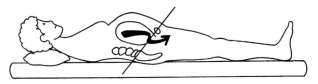

(b)

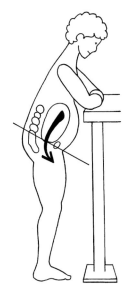

**Fig. 2.2**  Drive angle – (a) supine, (b) standing. Adapted from reference 12.

Frequent position changes in labor optimize the chance of a 'good fit' between the fetus and maternal pelvis (helping resolve occiput posterior position, asynclitism, and deflexion). Women often describe less pain when the fetus and pelvis are better aligned – an added benefit. Continuous movement (pelvic rocking, swaying, walking) results in continuing changes in the relationship of the pelvic bones to one another and the shape of the pelvis, which may serve to 'nudge' the fetus into a more favorable position.

No single position is optimal for all situations or for hours at a time. Therefore, the woman should be encouraged to move and try various positions and not to remain in one position when there is no apparent progress for long periods.

This book contains descriptions of various maternal positions and movements that may help in specific situations. See the Toolkit in Chapter 6 for a detailed description and discussion of each position and movement.

## MONITORING THE MOBILE WOMAN'S FETUS

There sometimes appears to be a trade-off between the advantages of maternal mobility and the presumed advantages of continuous electronic fetal monitoring (EFM) which usually requires the mother to remain lying in bed or semi-sitting. This trade-off can be resolved in a variety of ways. One way is to discontinue the routine practice of continuous EFM, because it carries virtually no benefit for the low-risk woman or baby, and some added dangers. For years it was assumed that continuous EFM improved newborn outcomes, but numerous scientific trials failed to confirm that assumption; in fact, these trials found that there were disadvantages associated with EFM, such as an increase in cesareans, with no improvement in outcomes[13].

### Auscultation

The findings of these trials led the professional organizations of obstetricians in the USA, Canada, and the UK to recommend other means of fetal surveillance.

Since 1988, the American College of Obstetricians and Gynecologists (ACOG) has supported alternatives to continuous electronic fetal monitoring for most women: 'It has been shown that intermittent auscultation at intervals of fifteen minutes during the first stage of labor and five minutes during the second stage is equivalent to continuous electronic fetal monitoring.'[14]

The Society of Obstetricians and Gynecologists of Canada (SOGC) is even more strongly supportive of intermittent auscultation:

> 'The preferred method of fetal health surveillance for low risk women during labour is intermittent fetal heart auscultation with a hand-held ultrasound Doppler.
>
> Such auscultation, for a full minute, should occur immediately after a contraction and be performed and documented every 30 minutes in the latent phase and every 15 to 30 minutes in the active phase of the first stage of labour and every five minutes in the second stage of labour once the patient has begun pushing.'[15]

The Royal College of Obstetricians and Gynaecologists also published a national policy on intrapartum surveillance for the UK in 1993: 'Auscultation is the method of choice for women at the normal end of the continuum of fetal risk.'[16]

## When electronic fetal monitoring is required: options to enhance maternal mobility

Despite these endorsements of intermittent auscultation, EFM has become well established and remains a method of monitoring in most hospitals in the USA, UK[17], and Canada. A high percentage still monitor continuously, even when the women are at low risk. Many doctors, nurses, and midwives who were trained in reading monitor tracings remain uneasy with auscultation. In many cases, the nurse or midwife may work in an institution where policies or doctors' orders require continuous EFM, and the women, despite the doctrines of informed consent and informed choice, have little say on this issue. There also are high-risk situations in which continuous EFM is called for. Is there anything that can be done to minimize the restriction to bed and the immobility that often accompany EFM?

The answer is yes.

## Continuous EFM

The woman does not have to remain in any single position or in bed. She may lie on her side, or sit up, or she may get out of bed and rock in a chair, stand and lean over the bed or a birth ball on the bed, sway or 'slow dance' (Fig. 2.3) with her partner beside the monitor, kneel, lunge, or even sit in the bath. (The Toolkit in Chapter 6 describes many of these techniques.)

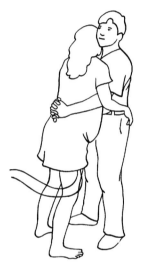

**Fig. 2.3**  Slow dancing with EFM.

Even if the fetal heart rate is easier to detect in one particular position, the woman should never be required to remain in that position for any longer than the time needed to document the heart rate. The woman's support person may be enlisted to hold the transducer in place (Fig. 2.4) or a washcloth may be placed between the transducer and its belt (Fig. 2.5) or mesh garment, so that it will not slip when the woman is in a standing, hands-and-knees, or other position. An internal scalp electrode usually has the advantage of not slipping out of place when the woman rolls over, kneels or squats (Fig. 2.6), as the external monitor may. However, the scalp electrode is more invasive than the external ultrasound transducer, requires ruptured mem-

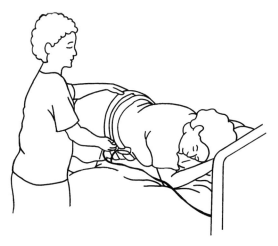

**Fig. 2.4**   Partner holding transducer in place.

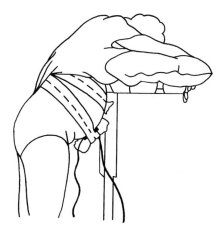

**Fig. 2.5**   Washcloth used to press transducer more firmly in place.

branes, and is more likely to promote maternal–fetal transmission of Human Immunodeficiency Virus (HIV) in an HIV positive mother. Because ultrasound devices are being improved, there is now less reliance on internal electronic fetal monitoring.

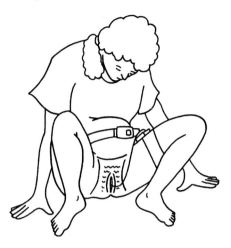

**Fig. 2.6**  Squatting with scalp electrode in place.

When an intrauterine pressure catheter (IUPC) is being used, a woman can also make use of upright positions, but it requires adjustment of the pressure gauge when the woman changes positions, in order to maintain accurate pressure readings. One should ask how important it is to record intrauterine pressure, and avoid it if there are no compelling clinical reasons to do so.

### Intermittent EFM

Some caregivers feel untrusting of their skills in auscultation, but do feel comfortable with intermittent EFM. This is a good example of a situation where 'informed choice' or 'informed consent' could guide the caregiver. If a woman is informed of the lack of benefit of continuous EFM, she might refuse it.

More likely, however, is that she will accept the option of intermittent electronic monitoring if her caregiver asks her to do so and explains his or her reasons. This usually means spending 15 or 20 minutes of each hour attached to the monitor, and being free to move about the rest of the time, sometimes with periodic auscultation between sessions on the monitor. She will be unencumbered and free to move about most of the time.

For women who prefer to spend part of their labor in the bath (Fig. 2.7), there are waterproof hand-held Doppler stethoscopes, but these are expensive and not available everywhere. Midwives who practice in out-of-hospital birth settings often use such devices. An ordinary ultrasound transducer that comes with the electronic fetal monitor can also be used while the woman is immersed in water. Check with your monitor manufacturer and your hospital's engineering department to be doubly sure, but the authors have frequently seen monitors used in the water and have been assured that there are no dangerous electronics in the transducer that can harm the woman or destroy the monitor when it is immersed in water (Chapter 7, p. 172).

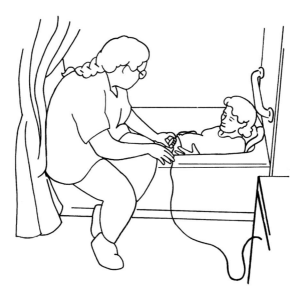

**Fig. 2.7**   Monitoring in bath.

## Telemetry

If the woman must be monitored continuously and the birth setting has an EFM telemetry unit, the woman may walk in or outside her room or sit in the bath or shower (Figs 2.8, 2.9). The telemetry unit either clips to the woman's robe or hangs over the side of the bath. Again, check with

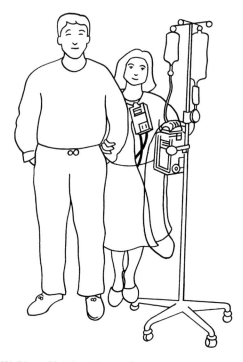

**Fig. 2.8**   Walking with telemetry monitor.

the monitor manufacturer and your hospital engineering department to be sure that monitoring in the water is safe with your particular device.

Considering the documented benefits of walking and hydrotherapy in speeding slow progress and pain reduction, telemetry may be the optimal choice of monitoring methods when continuous monitoring is called for. (For more on the prevention of dystocia through movement and ambulation see page 151, and for more on hydrotherapy see page 170.)

By implementing these ideas, it may be possible to avoid some of the problems caused by immobility and the horizontal position that usually accompany electronic fetal monitoring. These problems may include persistent occiput posterior position, less efficient contractions, supine hypotension (if the woman remains on her back), and excessive pain.

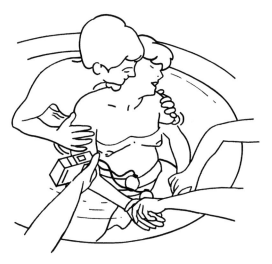

**Fig. 2.9** Telemetry in bath.

## TECHNIQUES TO ELICIT STRONGER CONTRACTIONS

The following techniques are associated with stronger or more frequent contractions.

- *Hydration.* Make sure that the woman is not dehydrated[8]. See page 66 for a discussion of hydration.
- *Movement and positioning.* If progress is slow, have the woman walk for half an hour, change positions frequently (about every half hour) and avoid the supine position.
- *Comforting touch,* such as stroking backrubs, hand-holding, etc., may increase endogenous oxytocin production (Fig. 2.10).
- *Nipple stimulation* done by either the woman or her partner can be used to stimulate contractions because it increases oxytocin production. The woman or her partner should start by stimulating one nipple, to see whether this will produce the desired effect. If not, both nipples may be stimulated. Contractions may become markedly longer and stronger so parents may need to be instructed to stop the nipple stimulation if contractions seem to become longer

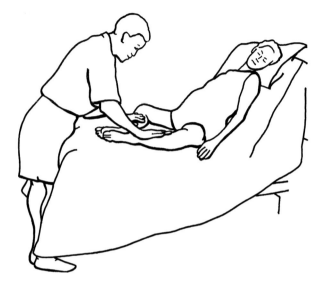

**Fig. 2.10**   Partner massaging woman's legs.

or stronger than is optimal for the fetus. See page 67 for references and more discussion.

- *Acupressure* may be used to augment contractions. See Chapter 7, page 174 for more information.
- *Warm compresses* or a hot water bottle placed on the fundus have been known to augment contractions. See Chapter 7, page 167, for information on the use of heat.

## CONCLUSION

In summary, this chapter describes practices that tend to prevent dystocia, with particular emphasis on minimizing maternal distress, promoting physiological measures that maintain progress, and encouraging movement and position changes by the woman.

## REFERENCES

1. O'Driscoll, K., Meagher, D. and Boylan, D. (1993) *Active Management of Labour*, 3rd edition. Mosby, London.

2. Crowther, C., Enkin, M., Keirse, M.J.N.C. and Brown, I. (1989) Monitoring the progress of labour. In: *Effective Care in Pregnancy and Childbirth*, vol. 2, Chalmers, I., Enkin, M., and Keirse, M.J.N.C. (eds). Oxford University Press, Oxford.

3. Odent, M. (1992) *The Nature of Birth and Breastfeeding*. Bergin & Garvey, Westport, CT.

4. Lederman, R.P., Lederman, E., Work, B.A. and McCann, D.S. (1981) Relationship of psychological factors in pregnancy to progress in labor. *Nurs. Res.* **25**, 94–8.

5. Lederman, E., Lederman, R.P., Work, B.A. and McCann, D.S. (1981) Maternal psychological and physiologic correlates of fetal-newborn health status. *Am. J. Obstet. Gynecol.* **139**, 956–60.

6. Newton, N. (1987) The fetus ejection reflex revisited. *Birth* **14**(2), 106–8.

7. Ludka, L.M. and Roberts, C.C. (1993) Eating and drinking in labor. *J. Nurs.-Midwif.* **38**(4), 199–207.

8. Sharp, D.A. (1997) Restriction of oral intake for women in labour. *Br. J. Midwif.* **5**(7), 408–12.

9. Berry, H. (1997) Feast or famine? Oral intake during labour: current evidence and practice. *Br. J. Midwif.* **5**(7), 413–17.

10. Roberts, J. (1989) Maternal position during the first stage of labour. In: *Effective Care in Pregnancy and Childbirth*, vol. 2, Chalmers, I., Enkin, M. and Keirse, M.J.N.C. (eds). Oxford University Press, Oxford.

11. Russell, J.G.B. (1969) Moulding of the pelvic outlet. *J. Obstet. Gynaecol. Br. Commonw.* **76**, 817–20.

12. Fenwick, L. and Simkin, P. (1987) Maternal positioning to treat dystocia. *Clin. Obstet. Gynecol.* **30**, 83–9.

13. Thacker, S.B. and Stroup, D.F. (1998) Continuous electronic fetal heart rate monitoring during labor. In: Neilson, J.P., Crowther, C.A., Hodnett, E.D. and Hofmeyr, G.J. (eds) Pregnancy and Childbirth Module of the Cochrane Database of Systematic Reviews (updated 2 December 1997). Available in the Cochrane Library. The Cochrane Collaboration, Oxford.

14. *Guidelines for Perinatal Care*, 2nd edition (1988) American Academy of Pediatrics and American College of Obstetricians and Gynecologists: Washington, DC, p. 67.

15. SOGC Policy Statement, No. 41, Part 1, October, 1995, p. 3.

16. Spencer, J.A.D. and Ward, R.H.T. (1993) *Intrapartum Fetal Surveillance*. RCOG Press, London.

17. Garcia, J., Redshaw, M., Fitzsimmons, B. and Keene, J. (1997) *First Class Delivery: A National Survey of Women's Views on Maternity Care*. Audit Commission, UK.

# Chapter 3
# Prolonged Pre-labor and Latent First Stage

## IS IT DYSTOCIA?

### When is a woman in labor?

This question, as fundamental as it may seem, is not easy to answer, and wide disagreement exists among experts. Two prominent obstetricians represent the extremes of opinion regarding the definition of labor. Emmanuel Friedman, who has profoundly influenced North American obstetricians regarding labor management, defines labor as follows: 'The onset of labor is defined simply as that time at which the patient first perceived regular uterine contractions. There is no way to distinguish true labor from false except by hindsight (when the contractions cease or when active dilation begins).'[1] At the other end of the spectrum, Kieran O'Driscoll and his colleagues in Ireland have a very precise definition of labor: painful contractions occurring at least every 10 minutes or closer, accompanied by at least one of the following: bloody mucous vaginal discharge; spontaneous rupture of the membranes; or complete cervical effacement[2].

These widely varying definitions of labor result in different management styles. According to Friedman, the latent phase in nulliparas averages 9 hours, and is considered 'prolonged' at 20 hours. O'Driscoll and colleagues would deny that a woman in Friedman's 'latent phase' is even in labor unless she exhibits their signs and symptoms mentioned above. Friedman suggests drug-induced rest for women with a prolonged latent phase, whereas O'Driscoll and colleagues do not admit her to the hospital or acknowledge any clinical significance to these contractions, regardless of what the women feel and think.

In this book, our definitions of labor are based on distinguishing between *progressing* and *non-progressing* contractions. *Progressing contractions* increase in one or more of the following measures: intensity, duration, and frequency. *Non-progressing contractions* remain the same over time. We are defining pre-labor as a period of regular, non-progressing contractions without an increase in cervical dilation, which may or may not continue without interruption into the latent phase. We define the latent phase of labor as the period beginning with continuous progressing contractions accompanied by cervical effacement and dilation and ending at 3 to 4 cm.

## The Woman Who Has Hours of Contractions Without Dilation

Sometimes it takes many hours, even days, of contractions before a woman's cervix dilates to 3 or 4 cm. To a great extent, the duration of pre-labor (sometimes referred to as 'false labor') or of latent first stage depends on the state of her cervix at the onset of contractions. If her cervix is unripe, uneffaced, and posterior, her pre-labor or latent phase will last longer than it would with a more favorable cervix.

Despite the differences in definitions of labor, most obstetric and midwifery textbook authors seem to agree that very little should be done to try to speed either pre-labor or the latent phase of labor in the absence of medical problems requiring imminent delivery[1,2,3,4]. Because most slow-starting labors eventually resolve into normal labor patterns, a diagnosis of dystocia or dysfunctional labor cannot accurately be made before the active phase[1]. Special supportive measures, in addition to those listed in Chapter 1, may be used to help the woman through the time necessary for her cervix to change. Chart 3.1 illustrates a step-by-step approach to the problem of a prolonged pre-labor or latent phase. Some of these same supportive measures apply when a woman is undergoing induction of labor, which sometimes lasts over several days.

**3**

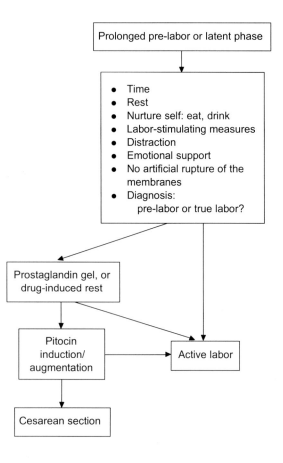

**Chart 3.1**

In this section we suggest ways to assess and meet the woman's support needs during a prolonged pre-labor or latent phase, especially when she describes or appears to experience more pain than women usually report at this degree of cervical dilation.

## THE SIX WAYS TO PROGRESS IN LABOR

Contractions without dilation are discouraging to the woman, who believes she is not making progress. She needs to understand that significant dilation can occur only when the cervix has already undergone preparatory changes. The caregiver should explain the reasons for pre-dilation (pre-labor) contractions in the context of the Six Ways to Progress. Although health care providers know these six ways, they often ignore the fact that when the cervix has not undergone the first three steps (ripening, effacement, and anterior movement), significant dilation (beyond 3 cm in the nullipara, more in the multipara) rarely occurs. There is a tendency among caregivers to minimize the importance of these three cervical changes when, in fact, progress in those areas is a very good sign and a necessary precursor to dilation. If such progress is ignored, an incorrect diagnosis of dysfunctional labor may be made before the woman is even in labor!

The following six steps must be accomplished in order for a baby to be born vaginally. For most women, the first three steps take place gradually, simultaneously, and almost unnoticed over a period of weeks before labor begins. *For a minority of women, however, hours or days of non-progressing pre-labor contractions are necessary to ready the cervix for dilation. Sometimes these contractions are intense enough to prevent sleep and the woman becomes discouraged and exhausted.*

Here are the six ways to progress:

(1)  The cervix moves from a posterior to an anterior position
(2)  The cervix ripens or softens
(3)  The cervix effaces
(4)  The cervix dilates
(5)  The fetal head rotates, flexes, and molds
(6)  The fetus descends and is born.

If the woman's cervix is not yet dilating, even though she is having contractions, she will need reassurance from her caregiver that these pre-labor contractions are accomplishing the important job of preparing her cervix to dilate. She *is* making necessary progress. Before dilation begins, support measures should focus on educating the woman about the six ways to progress, encouraging her to engage in distracting activities, helping her to accept the slow progress of early labor as a normal variation, preventing exhaustion, meeting her nutritional needs, and keeping her comfortable.

Rotation, flexion, molding, and descent of the fetal head take place in active labor and second stage. These will be discussed in Chapters 4 and 5.

## SUPPORT MEASURES FOR WOMEN WHO ARE AT HOME IN PRE-LABOR AND LATENT PHASE

**3**

While most women remain at home during this phase, some will come to the hospital and some will call for phone advice. It helps if they have been taught in advance or given a list of ways to cope with early labor. In the absence of medical contraindications, these suggestions will help the woman maintain normal progress and confidence:

- She should continue normal activities – rest (even if she cannot sleep) at night, do pleasant distracting activities during the day – for as long as possible, but avoid overexertion.

- She should have her partner or a friend or relative remain with her.

- If it is night time and the woman can rest, she should lie down or relax in the tub. (Please note: immersion in water in early labor may temporarily stop contractions and give the woman some rest[5]. This is an advantage if she needs rest, but a disadvantage if it is important that her labor progresses.)

- If she is unable to rest, or it is daytime, she should try distraction measures, such as:
  - going for a walk or having someone take her for a drive
  - visiting with friends or family
  - going to a movie or other entertainment, shopping
  - preparing meals for after the birth
  - baking bread
  - preparing the baby's clothing, bedding

- ○ watching videotapes, TV
- ○ doing a 'project' – sorting photos, writing in a journal, cleaning a closet, drawing or painting
- ○ playing games, and others

● She should eat when hungry, unless she knows she is having a cesarean section (e.g. because of a herpes lesion, a complicated presentation, or other pre-existing condition). Best choices are easily digested complex carbohydrates (starchy foods, fruits and vegetables). She should avoid greasy or highly spiced foods.

● She should drink to thirst. Water, broth, fruit juice, caffeine-free teas, or electrolyte-balanced beverages are good choices.

● She should begin using labor coping techniques during her contractions when distraction is no longer possible (when she cannot walk through or talk through her contractions without pausing at the peaks). Such techniques as relaxation and self-calming, slow breathing (sighing), and attention-focusing are appropriate at this time.

● She should periodically time four or five consecutive contractions for duration, frequency, and interval to determine if her contractions are progressing. She should be given guidelines on when to come to the hospital (including guidelines on ruptured membranes).

● Some women, having no idea of what to expect from early labor, 'over-react', that is, they are preoccupied with every contraction, and they may rush to use learned coping techniques that are more appropriate for active labor. They often expect to be 5 or 6 cm dilated when they are first checked and are crushed when they are examined and found to be only 1 to 2 cm! They do not see how they are going to cope with the more intense contractions to come. A woman in this situation needs a chance to express her disappointment. The caregiver can help by acknowledging her disappointment, giving her some suggestions to reduce the intensity of the contractions, and proceed to calm and relax her. She 'will need help to get her head back where her cervix is'[6].

If a woman arrives at the hospital earlier than necessary, she is often encouraged to return home. The manner in which this is handled can make her feel either more confident, knowledgeable, and willing to go home, or ashamed, angry, or afraid to leave the hospital. If the above measures are followed, the former is more likely.

## SOME REASONS FOR EXCESSIVE PAIN AND DURATION OF PRE-LABOR OR LATENT PHASE

For some women, pre-labor or latent phase is extremely painful and prolonged for a variety of reasons:

### Physical reasons

- Oxytocin-induced contractions are sometimes painful and debilitating, especially when a woman is having contractions every 2 or 3 minutes and her cervix is only 1 or 2 cm dilated.
- Policies or practices that restrict the woman to bed. Reasons for such a policy include ruptured membranes (see page 36); continuous electronic fetal monitoring (see page 19); and pregnancy-induced hypertension (see page 36). In many cases, restriction to bed is not required, but no one encourages the woman to get out of bed.
- A scarred cervix from previous surgery (for example, cryosurgery, cone biopsy) may increase the resistance of the cervix to effacement and the first few centimeters of dilation. Contractions of great intensity for many hours or days may be required to overcome this resistance after which dilation.
- Occiput posterior position of the fetus.

### Psychological reasons

- Extreme fear, anxiety, loneliness, stress, or anger may lead to a build-up of catecholamines and a resulting slowdown in progress (see page 13). Women who are unsupported emotionally, or have experienced previous difficult childbirths, traumatic experiences such as child abuse, substance abuse, multiple hospitalizations, or domestic violence may find early labor unexpectedly painful.
- Exhaustion, discouragement, and feelings of hopelessness result from a long pre-labor or latent phase. The woman's coping ability diminishes and her pain worsens as time goes on without apparent progress.

It may be helpful to ask the woman how she feels emotionally during latent labor. Her answer may assist the caregiver in diagnosing emotional distress. Between contractions, questions such as 'what was going through your mind during that contraction?' or 'how are you feeling right now?' or 'why do you think this labor is going slowly right now?' may reveal that the mother is distressed or worried over specific concerns. Knowing these concerns will help the caregiver support the woman emotionally. See Chapter 7, pages 179–82, for more on how to help an emotionally distressed woman.

The next section offers suggestions to improve labor progress or reduce discomfort in early labor. Of course, if fetal distress, macrosomia, malpresentation, inadequate contractions, or other complications are diagnosed, the supportive measures will have to be tailored to the situation.

**3**

## TROUBLESHOOTING MEASURES FOR PAINFUL PROLONGED PRE-LABOR OR LATENT PHASE

- Follow the general measures for early labor as appropriate (page 11).

- For the pain and discouragement that may accompany some labor inductions or a scarred cervix, reassure the woman that under these circumstances early labor is more challenging, but it does not mean that active labor will be abnormal.

- Try not to contribute to her self-doubt or worries by suggesting that something is wrong. (Patients with prolonged latent phase are no more prone to develop subsequent labor aberrations than those with normal latent phases; at the same time, they are not immune to other problems, of course[7].)

- If she is discouraged over slow dilation or non-progressing contractions, remind the woman that before her cervix can dilate, it must move forward, ripen, and efface – each of which is a positive sign of progress. Be sure to disclose any progress in these areas to her whenever you check her cervix. See Six Ways to Progress on page 31.

- Avoid the term 'false labor' because it implies that her contractions are somehow 'unreal' and that because her cervix is not dilating, the contractions are not accomplishing anything significant. In fact, these pre-labor contractions are preparing the cervix for dilation. Such implications are most discouraging to the woman who is experiencing them.

- Encourage her to seek and use those positions or movements that she finds more comfortable. See 'Monitoring the mobile woman's fetus,' page 18, for suggestions on monitoring during induced labor.

- Offer a bath or shower or massage as a temporary relaxer and pain reliever.

- A drug-induced rest with a pain reliever may be an appropriate choice.

*Note:* If at all possible, do not restrict the woman to bed. Before restricting a woman with ruptured membranes to bed (which is a requirement in many hospitals even if the fetal head is engaged) the caregiver might auscultate the fetal heart and assess fetal movement with the woman in an upright position. Sometimes the upright position may actually protect against prolapsed cord, as gravity may keep the head applied to the cervix, thus preventing the cord from slipping through.

- Many caregivers, especially in North America, restrict the woman with pregnancy-induced hypertension to bed in late pregnancy and in labor, because blood pressure is usually lowered while a woman lies on her left side. Whether such treatment has resulted in improved outcomes or less progression of pre-eclampsia is not known[8]. The topic requires further study. However, if you are caring for a woman who is in bed with pregnancy-induced hypertension, you can explain why left-sided bedrest is being asked of her (while acknowledging the lack of study in this area). Help her focus on comfort measures that she can use while in bed. Relaxation, breathing patterns, vocalization, guided imagery, visualizations, other attention-focusing measures, and massage of her back or feet may help. In addition, if limited walking is acceptable, she may walk to and from the bathroom, to use the shower or tub (both of which frequently lower high blood pressure).

- Assess the woman's emotional state during early labor and, if she is distressed, try appropriate measures to help improve her emotional state. See the Toolkit, Chapter 7, pages 179–82.

- For exhaustion, discouragement, and hopelessness, you can raise her spirits by suggesting a change: have her wash her face, comb her hair, brush her teeth, take a walk, play some upbeat music. This is especially effective as the sun comes up after a long night with little progress.

- Have a good talk with her and her partner, encouraging them to express their feelings. Acknowledge and validate their feelings of frustration, discouragement, fatigue, or even anger at the staff for not 'doing something' to correct the problem. She may benefit from a good cry, followed by a pep talk and perhaps a visit from a friend or family member who is rested and optimistic.

## MEASURES TO ALLEVIATE PAINFUL IRREGULAR NON-DILATING CONTRACTIONS IN PRE-LABOR OR LATENT PHASE

**3**

If early contractions are painful and irregular with little or no progress in dilation, it makes sense to consider persistent asynclitism or another unfavorable fetal position, such as occiput posterior (Figs 3.1a, b, 3.2, 3.3). Labor normally begins with the fetal head in asynclitism, (the head is angled so that one of the parietal bones, rather than the vertex, presents at the pelvic inlet). This facilitates passage of the fetal head through the pelvic inlet, and then the head usually shifts into synclitism so that the vertex presents as the head descends further. However,

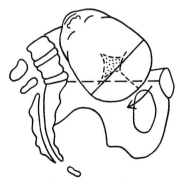

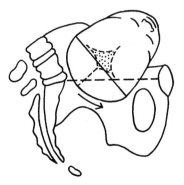

**Fig. 3.1a** Posterior asynclitism.     **Fig. 3.1b** Anterior asynclitism.

sometimes the asynclitism persists and, if so, it can keep the fetus from rotating and descending[9]. Without descent, the head may not be well applied to the cervix and contractions often become irregular and ineffective. At this stage of labor, it is difficult or impossible (and not considered very clinically important) to assess the angle and position of the fetal head. However, if contractions are irregular and ineffective for a long time, position changes and movements may correct the problem and improve the contraction pattern.

---

*Note regarding artificial rupture of the membranes (AROM) with a malpositioned fetus*

AROM is often done in an attempt to speed a slow labor. However, when the fetus is occiput posterior, occiput transverse, or asynclitic, AROM may have no benefit, or may even interfere with progress. The randomized controlled trials of amniotomy have investigated effects of routine early amniotomy only on spontaneous labor, but not on dystotic labor[10]. The question remains as to whether rupturing membranes is beneficial for a delay in active labor in which a malposition, cephalo-pelvic disproportion (CPD), or macrosomia is present[11]. The arguments against amniotomy for dystocia are based on concerns over the risks (prolapsed cord, infection), and over the loss of the benefits of the forewaters, which are thought to provide some protection and maneuvering space for the fetal head. When the forewaters are removed, the malpositioned fetus may be subjected to uneven head compression, more molding, and a greater chance of operative delivery than would otherwise occur. Furthermore, it is not known whether the malposition is more likely to self-correct with or without intact membranes. Without clear evidence of benefit, these potential risks remain a concern. If stronger contractions are needed, other methods to intensify contractions might be tried first. These include relatively benign measures, such as position changes and movement, acupressure, and nipple stimulation (see Toolkit, Chapters 6 and 7, and p. 67), any of which may render AROM or intravenous oxytocin unnecessary.

---

If the woman is having her first baby or has good abdominal muscle tone, having her lean forward often moves the fetus's center of gravity forward, encouraging its head to pivot into a more favorable position (Figs 3.4, 3.5). This may even out or increase the head-to-cervix force, leading to more regular, more effective contractions.

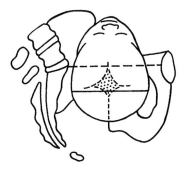

**Fig. 3.2** Synclitism.

3

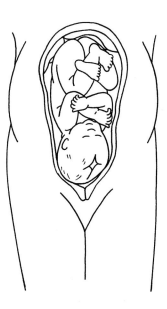

**Fig. 3.3** Right occiput posterior – abdominal view.

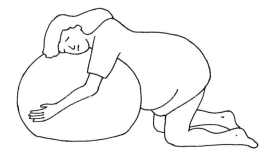

**Fig. 3.4** Kneeling with a ball.

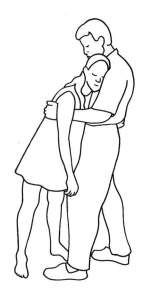

**Fig. 3.5** Standing leaning on partner.

The open knee–chest position may take advantage of gravity to allow the fetus to 'back out' of the woman's pelvis and descend again in a more favorable position.

El Halta[12], an American midwife, teaches the open knee–chest position for specific symptoms in pre-labor or the latent phase, when there is a long period of frequent, irregular and brief uterine contractions, usually accompanied by severe persistent backache, but resulting in little or no dilation. El Halta's experience is that such a contraction pattern is associated with an occiput posterior position. She instructs the woman to spend 30 to 45 minutes in an open knee–chest position, that is, her hips are flexed to an angle greater than $90°$ (Fig. 3.6).

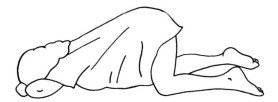

**Fig. 3.6**  Open knee–chest position.

The open knee–chest position tilts the pelvis forward enough for the optimal gravity effect in encouraging the fetal head out of the pelvis, and may allow the head to reposition more favorably before re-entering the pelvis. (By contrast, a 'closed knee–chest position' would mean that the woman's hips and knees are flexed so that her thighs are beneath her abdomen. This gives less room for the fetus to move out of the pelvis and less gravity effect.)

If the woman's abdominal muscle tone is poor and her abdomen is pendulous, suggest that she try a semi-sitting position (Fig. 3.7). Having her 'lean back' in this way may move the fetus's center of gravity toward her back, thus angling its head into a more synclitic position. This allows the head to put more pressure on the cervix, and may lead to more regular, more effective contractions.

King suggests abdominal lifting (Fig. 3.8) with a pelvic tilt during contractions at any time in labor if the woman has back pain in association with pendulous abdominal muscles, a short waist, a previous back injury, or an occiput posterior baby. Abdominal lifting, when it works well, realigns the angle between the baby's torso and the pelvic

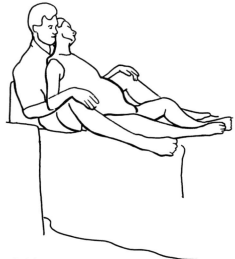

**Fig. 3.7**   Semi-sitting.

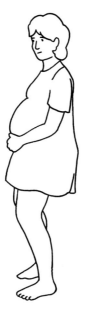

**Fig. 3.8**   Abdominal lifting.

inlet. The contractions then become more efficient in pressing the baby's head onto the cervix. See 'Toolkit,' Chapter 6, page 160 for specific instructions[13].

## CONCLUSION

Prolonged pre-labor and the latent phase of labor in themselves rarely indicate a complication, although they are discouraging and exhausting for the woman. Suggestions are given for coping with the discouragement, and early measures to correct possible fetal malposition. Most of the measures suggested here are well tolerated or favored by women, but if a woman finds them distressing or uncomfortable, she should be encouraged to do what she finds most helpful.

**3**

## REFERENCES

1. Friedman, E.A. (1993) Dysfunctional labor. In: *Management of Labor*, Cohen, W.R. and Friedman, E.A. (eds). University Park Press, Baltimore, p. 17.
2. O'Driscoll, K., Meagher, D. and Boylan, P. (1993) *Active Management of Labour*, 3rd edition. Baillière Tindall, London.
3. Davis, E. (1997) *Heart and Hands: A Midwife's Guide to Pregnancy and Birth*, 3rd edition. Celestial Arts, Berkeley.
4. Varney, H. (1997) *Varney's Midwifery*, 3rd edition. Jones and Bartlett Publishers, Boston.
5. Eriksson, M., Mattsson, L.A. and Ladfors, L. (1997) Early or late bath during the first stage of labour: a randomized study of 200 women. *Midwifery* **13(3)**, 146–8.
6. Wilf, R. (1980) Personal communication.
7. Friedman, E.A. (1978) *Labor: Clinical Evaluation and Management*, 2nd edition. Appleton Century Crofts, New York, p. 78.
8. Enkin, M., Keirse, M.J.N.C., Renfrew, M. and Neilson, J. (1995) Hypertension in pregnancy. In: *A Guide to Effective Care in Pregnancy and Childbirth*, 2nd edition. Oxford University Press, Oxford.
9. Oxorn, H. (1980) *Oxorn–Foote Human Labour and Birth*, 4th edition. Appleton Century Crofts, New York.
10. Fraser, W.D., Krauss, I., Brisson-Carrol, G., Thornton, J. and Breart, G. (1998) Amniotomy to shorten spontaneous labor. In: *Pregnancy and Childbirth Module of the Cochrane Database of Systematic Reviews* (updated quarterly). Available in the Cochrane Library (database on disk and CD-ROM). The Cochrane Collaboration, Issue 2. Oxford Update Software.
11. Keirse, M.J.N.C. (1989) Augmentation of labour. In: *Effective Care in*

*Pregnancy and Childbirth*, vol. 2, Chalmers, I., Enkin, M. and Keirse, M.J.N.C. (eds). Oxford University Press, Oxford.

12. El Halta, V. (1995) Posterior labor: A pain in the back. *Midwif. Today* **36**, 19–21.

13. King, J.M. (1993) *Back Labor No More!! What Every Woman Should Know Before Labor.* Plenary Systems, Dallas.

Chapter 4

# Prolonged Active Phase of Labor

**4**

## WHAT IS PROLONGED ACTIVE LABOR?

The active phase of labor (or active labor) usually refers to cervical
dilation greater than 3 cm accompanied by progressing contractions,
that is, contractions that are becoming longer, stronger and more
frequent. It should be noted that multiparas sometimes reach 3, 4 or
even 5 cm of dilation without progressing contractions. They are not in
labor until they begin having progressing contractions and their cervices dilate further with contractions.

The term *prolonged active labor* refers to an insufficient rate of dilation after active labor has been diagnosed. The diagnosis of 'insufficient rate of progress' varies: less than 1 cm per hour for at least two
hours after labor progress has been well established[1]; less than 1.2 cm
per hour in a primigravida and less than 1.5 cm per hour in a multipara[2]; longer than 12 hours from 4 cm to complete dilation (which
translates to 0.5 cm per hour)[3,4,5].

## CHARACTERISTICS OF PROLONGED ACTIVE LABOR

- The contractions slow down, that is, they become less intense,
  shorter in duration, and/or less frequent, or
- Contractions take on a quality of sameness, neither progressing nor
  slowing down.
- The woman continues coping in the same way for hours, or finds
  labor easier to manage.
- On a vaginal exam, the cervix is unchanged.

Clinical management of prolonged active labor varies, depending on
the caregiver's philosophy and the woman's wishes, for example:

- The most common approach, once the diagnosis has been made, is to rupture the membranes (if that has not already been done) and start incremental doses of intravenous oxytocin. If these measures are unsuccessful in stimulating progress, a cesarean delivery is performed[6].

- In the active management of labor protocol[1], as practiced at the National Maternity Hospital in Dublin and elsewhere, the membranes are ruptured as soon as labor is diagnosed. If dilation is less than 1 cm per hour for two hours at any time after labor is diagnosed (regardless of cervical dilation), high doses of oxytocin are administered incrementally until a rate of at least 1 cm per hour is achieved.

- With midwifery care or a low intervention model of obstetric care, the caregiver assesses the rate of dilation, but perceives a slow rate of dilation in the active phase as an indication for evaluation rather than medical intervention. The caregiver is likely to make broader allowances for individual variations in progress of dilation, taking into account fetal and maternal tolerance of the delay and assessing signs of progress other than dilation, such as rotation of the fetal head, which is often a necessary precursor to further progress. (See Chapter 3, page 31, 'Six Ways to Progress in Labor'.) Such an approach relies on preventive measures, and time, patience, support, and primary interventions such as those offered in this book. The goals are to support the woman through the delay and encourage labor progress[4,7]. Oxytocin and artificial rupture of the membranes are reserved for later use if necessary.

## POSSIBLE CAUSES OF PROLONGED ACTIVE LABOR

Slowing or arrest of dilation in the active phase may sometimes be prevented or corrected by use of simple, low-cost, early interventions that carry little or no known risk. If they are not successful, then the woman will need the more powerful and complex obstetric interventions that are more expensive and are associated with more potential risks. Chart 4.1 illustrates a step-by-step approach to the problem of a prolonged active phase of labor.

The choice of intervention depends on the apparent cause of the problem. The most common causes of prolonged active labor are:

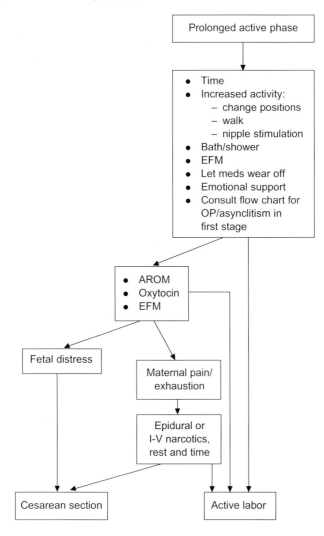

**4**

**Chart 4.1**

- Malpositions: occiput posterior, persistent occiput transverse position, or persistent asynclitism.
- Macrosomia (a large fetus) or cephalo-pelvic disproportion (CPD – a poor fit between the fetal head and maternal pelvis). Macrosomia is sometimes associated with CPD, but CPD more often takes place when an average or relatively small fetal head does not fit because of a discrepancy between the shape, position or attitude of the head and the dimensions of the pelvis.
- Inadequate intensity of contractions.
- Persistent cervical lip.
- 'Emotional dystocia': fear, anxiety, tension, or hostility.
- Maternal exhaustion, dehydration.
- Maternal physical factors: short waist, severe lumbar lordosis (especially if combined with a lack of mobility in the lumbar spine), or a pendulous abdomen, due to lack of abdominal muscle tone[8].
- Combination of etiologies or unknown etiology.

Sometimes the delay in progress results from a combination of the above, for example, a persistent malposition associated with a large baby, maternal fear or exhaustion, and inadequate contractions. Sometimes the cause is unclear. In such cases, the contractions appear adequate, fetal position appears favorable, fetal size seems average, and the woman appears to be coping well, but progress in dilation is slow. Patience and trial and error, using a number of the measures discussed in this chapter, may result in greater progress without anyone figuring out exactly what the problem is. It may be a subtle undetectable variation in position or some other factor that may be corrected with the passage of time and a variety of movements and comfort measures.

## MALPOSITION, MACROSOMIA AND CEPHALO-PELVIC DISPROPORTION (CPD)

With information gained from observations of abdominal shape, abdominal palpation, the woman's symptoms, the contraction pattern, internal examination of the suture lines of the fetal skull, the caregiver might suspect fetal malposition, macrosomia, or cephalo-pelvic disproportion (CPD). Even if the specific etiology is not clear, however, the primary interventions for all of these conditions are very similar, so

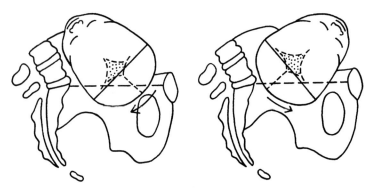

**Fig. 4.1**   Posterior asynclitism.          **Fig. 4.2**   Anterior asynclitism.

a trial and error approach is usually acceptable. These interventions are grouped in this section.

At the onset of labor, most fetuses are normally in an asynclitic occiput transverse (OT) or occiput anterior (OA) position (Figs 4.1 and 4.2). This means the fetal head is angled so that one parietal bone enters the pelvis first. The fetal biparietal diameter is not parallel to the plane of the inlet of the pelvis. In synclitism, the fetal biparietal diameter is parallel to the plane of the inlet. See Fig. 4.3. With contractions, the head usually pivots into synclitism as it descends. Only if asynclitism is persistent, that is, remaining when the fetus is at a low station, does it slow labor progress.

The occiput posterior (OP) position occurs in 15–30% of all labors,

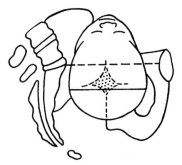

**Fig. 4.3**   Synclitism.

and is more common in primigravidas. A 'dip' in the supine woman's abdomen at the level of the umbilicus is a sign of an OP fetus[9]. Most OP fetuses rotate spontaneously by late first stage. Contractions, gravity, resilience of the muscles in the pelvis, the woman's position and movement, and other forces encourage rotation of the fetal head. OP and OT positions (Figs 4.4 and 4.5) and asynclitism usually

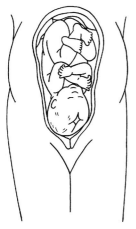

**Fig. 4.4** Right occiput posterior seen from front.

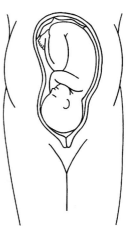

**Fig. 4.5** Left occiput transverse fetus.

become problems if they persist, although with time, if the woman's pelvis is roomy enough, the fetus may be born in those positions.

Many cases of 'suspected CPD' actually involve fetuses who are subtly malpositioned (asynclitic, occiput posterior, deflexed chin). In other words, the head is not too large, but the way it is positioned makes for a poor fit. The head may fit well once the malposition has been resolved, but accomplishing this may require extra time, support, and specific efforts by the woman and staff. As long as the fetus and woman can tolerate it, the passage of time is often all that is necessary either to solve the problem or, if the problem does not resolve, to confirm the diagnosis of arrest of active labor.

## Reasons for delayed progress

When rotation or improved alignment is needed, it makes sense that labor will take more time than when the fetus is ideally positioned. Dilation may begin later or take longer, because the pressure of the fetal head or forewaters on the cervix, which normally enhances dilation, may be uneven or generally reduced. Descent may also be delayed until the fetal head rotates, flexes, or aligns with the plane of the pelvis.

One should always suspect a malposition, asynclitism, cephalo-pelvic disproportion, or macrosomia if:

- contractions are irregular (varying in intensity and duration in an unpredictable way)
- contractions 'couple' (two or three close together, followed by a relatively long interval)
- contractions 'space out' or slow down in active labor
- the woman complains of back pain that may or may not go away between contractions
- labor progress plateaus in active labor
- the woman has an uncontrollable urge to push long before dilation is complete.

## Artificial rupture of the membranes

When there is a delay in active labor, caregivers often rupture the membranes to speed it up. There is some concern over the wisdom of such a practice when the fetus is malpositioned[6]. See page 38 in Chapter 3 for further explanation.

## Specific measures to address and correct problems associated with malposition, cephalo-pelvic disproportion, and macrosomia

Besides those discussed in this chapter, see Chapter 1 for general measures to aid labor progress, and Chapter 7, page 182, for back pain interventions and devices.

## MATERNAL POSITIONS AND MOVEMENTS FOR SUSPECTED OCCIPUT POSTERIOR, PERSISTENT OCCIPUT TRANSVERSE, ASYNCLITISM, CEPHALO-PELVIC DISPROPORTION OR MACROSOMIA IN ACTIVE LABOR

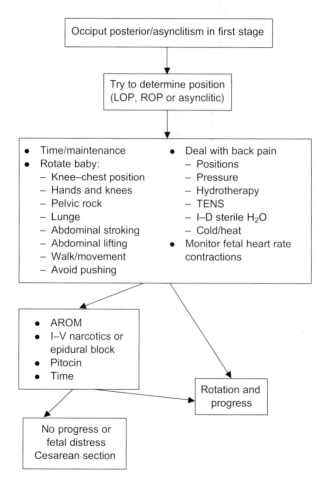

**Chart 4.2**

Chart 4.2 illustrates a step-by-step approach to be used when an occiput posterior or asynclitism is suspected. Besides use of a variety of maternal positions (illustrated in this section), helping the woman to deal with back pain (described in Chapter 7) is an important element in her care.

Maternal positions and movements alter the forces of gravity and the various pressures on the uterus and pelvic joints. The position of the fetus is influenced by these changing forces. (See Chapter 6 for more information on each position and movement.)

## Forward-leaning positions

Figures 4.6–4.16 show forward leaning positions that may aid fetal repositioning.

See pages 133–41 for an explanation of how these positions may correct some problems of a 'poor fit' between fetus and maternal pelvis.

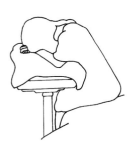

**Fig. 4.6**  Sitting leaning on a tray table.

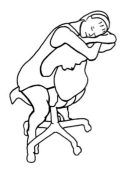

**Fig. 4.7**  Straddling a chair.

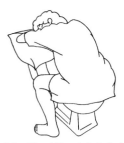

**Fig. 4.8**  Straddling toilet, facing backwards.

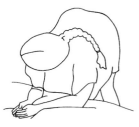

**Fig. 4.9**  Standing, leaning on bed.

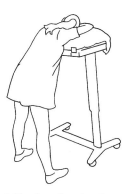

**Fig. 4.10** Standing, leaning on a tray table.

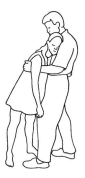

**Fig. 4.11** Standing, leaning forward on partner.

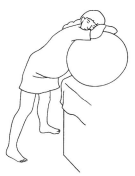

**Fig. 4.12** Standing, leaning on ball.

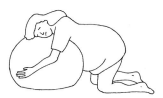

**Fig. 4.13** Kneeling with a ball.

**4**

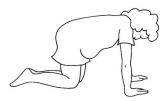

**Fig. 4.14** Hands and knees.

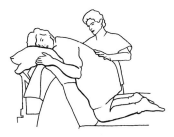

**Fig. 4.15** Kneeling over bed back.

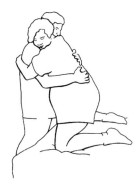

**Fig. 4.16** Kneeling, partner support.

## Sidelying positions

When the fetus is thought to be occiput posterior (OP), the woman using 'pure sidelying' should lie on the side *toward* which the occiput is already directed, or baby's back 'toward bed', see Figs 4.17 and 4.18. But, if she is semi-prone, she should lie on the side *opposite* the direction of the occiput (fetal back 'toward ceiling', Fig. 4.19).

See pages 59 and 126–9 for an explanation of how sidelying may correct some problems of a 'poor fit' between fetus and maternal pelvis.

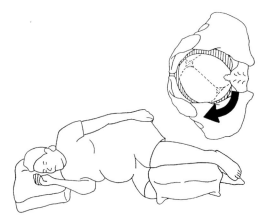

**Fig. 4.17** Woman in pure sidelying on the 'correct' side, with fetal back 'toward the bed'. If fetus is ROP, woman lies on her right side. Gravity pulls fetal head and trunk towards ROT.

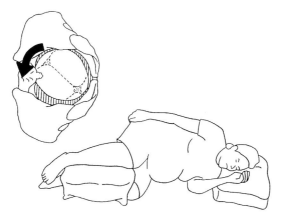

**Fig. 4.18** Woman in pure sidelying on the 'wrong' (left) side for an ROP fetus. Fetal back is toward the ceiling. Gravity pulls fetal occiput and trunk toward direct OP.

**4**

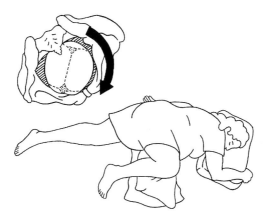

**Fig. 4.19** Woman semi-prone on the 'correct side' – with fetal back 'toward the ceiling'. If fetus is ROP, the semi-prone woman lies on her left side. Gravity pulls fetal occiput and trunk toward ROT, then ROA.

## Asymmetrical positions and movements

Asymmetrical positions and movements (Figs 4.20–4.24) enlarge the pelvis on the side where the leg is raised and slightly alter the internal shape of the pelvis. This may allow more space where it is needed for rotation. To master the technique of the lunge, please see the instructions in Chapter 6, page 154, before teaching it to the woman in labor.

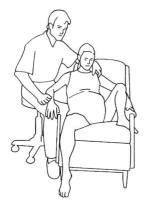

**Fig. 4.20**   Sitting with one leg elevated.

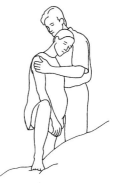

**Fig. 4.21**   Standing with one leg elevated.

(a)

(b)

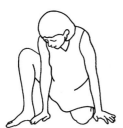

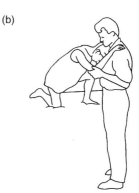

**Fig. 4.22**   (a) Asymmetrical kneeling, (b) asymmetrical kneeling, leaning on partner.

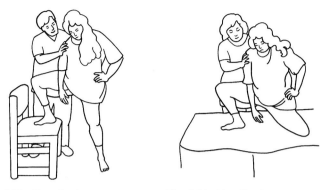

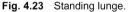
**Fig. 4.23** Standing lunge.

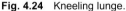
**Fig. 4.24** Kneeling lunge.

---

***Note regarding supine and semi-sitting positions for occiput posterior***

When a woman is fully supine or semi-sitting, gravity encourages the trunk of the OP fetus to lie next to the woman's spine, increasing the chances of supine hypotension, but also minimizing the likelihood of rotation to OA. These positions also increase the pressure of the fetal occiput against the woman's sacrum, thus worsening her back pain (Fig. 4.25a). There is a much greater likelihood of rotation, and less back pain when the woman sits upright or leans forward[9,10] (Fig. 4.25b).

When a woman is supine, the head of an occiput posterior fetus is directed more toward the pubic bone during contractions (Fig. 4.26a). When the woman is upright, the uterus, tilting forward, directs the fetal head into the pelvic basin (Fig. 4.26b).

---

**4**

(a)

(b)

**Fig. 4.25** (a) Woman reclining. Weight of uterus rests on her spine. Adapted from reference 10. (b) Woman upright. Fundus tilts forward. Adapted from reference 10.

(a) (b)

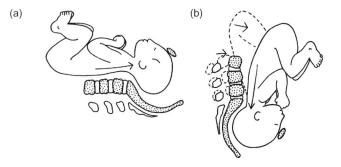

**Fig. 4.26** (a) Woman reclining. Head of OP fetus directed toward pubic bone. Adapted from reference 10. (b) Woman upright. Head directed into pelvic basin. Adapted from reference 10.

## Abdominal lifting

To improve the alignment of the fetal trunk and head with the axis of the birth canal, the woman places her hands beneath her abdomen and during contractions lifts her abdomen while tilting her pelvis and bending her knees[8] (Fig. 4.27). See Chapter 6, page 160, for complete instructions on abdominal lifting.

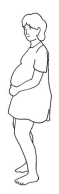

**Fig. 4.27** Abdominal lifting.

## AN UNCONTROLLABLE PREMATURE URGE TO PUSH

An uncontrollable, almost convulsive urge to push during active labor sometimes accompanies an OP position, especially when the fetus is deeply engaged. The caregiver is faced with the question of whether the woman should push or not (Chart 4.3). On the one hand, with a prolonged active phase and an OP fetus, her pushing might lead to a swollen cervix or even a torn cervix, and no further progress. On the other hand, it is sometimes impossible for the woman to control this urge.

A change of position to hands and knees (Fig. 4.28), semi-prone (exaggerated Sims, Fig. 4.29) or open knee–chest (Fig. 4.30), may relieve the urge to push by using gravity to move the head away from the cervix and ease pressure on the posterior vaginal wall (which seems to be the factor responsible for the urge to push). Manual repositioning of the fetal head (page 108) may also help.

**4**

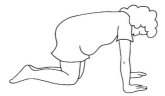

**Fig. 4.28** Hands and knees.

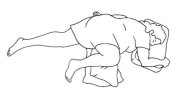

**Fig. 4.29** Semi-prone, lower arm back.

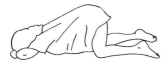

**Fig. 4.30** Open knee–chest position.

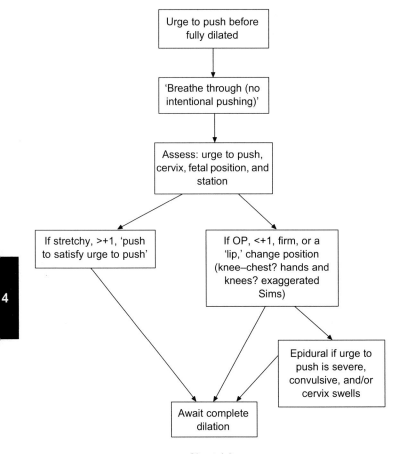

**Chart 4.3**

## HYDROTHERAPY (BATHS AND SHOWERS: FIGS 4.31 AND 4.32)

Buoyancy, hydrostatic pressure, warmth, skin stimulation, and other factors induce relaxation, temporarily reduce pain awareness, and may speed progress in active labor. For guidelines on the use of hydrotherapy, see Chapter 7, page 188.

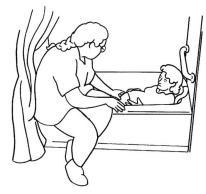

**Fig. 4.31** A bath to speed progress in active labor.

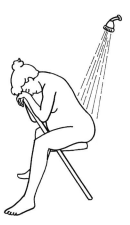

**4**

**Fig. 4.32** A shower to speed progress in active labor.

## REST

Fatigue or exhaustion, especially if the woman is upset or afraid, is a major concern for women experiencing long labors. Massage, music, aromatherapy, guided imagery, a bath or whatever she finds soothing may relax her and help her accept the slow pace of her labor. A patient and empathic caregiver conveys feelings of well-being and can ease the worry.

## Positions for tired women

The positions shown in Figs 4.33–4.36 may be useful for tired women. Also see Chapter 1 for general measures to maintain labor progress.

(a)                                              (b)

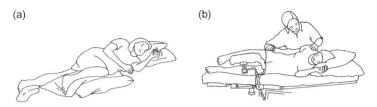

**Fig. 4.33**   (a) Semi-prone, lower arm forward, (b) lateral with leg support.

**4**

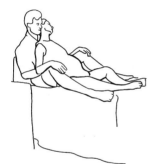

**Fig. 4.34**   Semi-sitting.

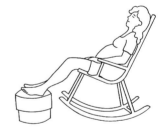

**Fig. 4.35**   Sitting in a rocking chair.

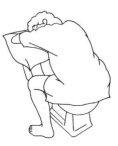

**Fig. 4.36**   Sitting backward on toilet.

# IF CONTRACTIONS ARE INADEQUATE

If contractions seem to be of inadequate intensity, consider whether immobility, medication, dehydration, or emotional factors could be contributing factors.

## Immobility

Has the woman been in one position for over half an hour? Changing her position may trigger stronger contractions, either by shifting the fetus's weight or by improving circulation to the uterus. Upright positions and movements, including walking, may intensify contractions. The supine position, by contrast, is correlated with weaker contractions, when compared with other positions[11]. The supine position is also a contributor to supine hypotension (low maternal blood pressure and decreased placental blood flow).

Unfortunately, few trials have been conducted on the effects of walking or position changes as an intervention to correct labor dystocia. The trials of ambulation in normal labor have shown no harm to women in normal labor who walk[12]. One large trial found that, when asked, 99% of the women who had been assigned to walk in labor (and did so) said they would choose to do so again[12]. Therefore, a lack of harm and high acceptance by women may be justification enough to encourage walking and position changes in labor.

## Medication

Narcotic analgesia received early in labor may temporarily reduce the intensity of the woman's contractions. Simply allowing medications to wear off may lead to stronger contractions, although the woman may find this intolerable.

Epidurals are associated with dystocia, but there is not a proven cause-and-effect relationship. There is controversy as to whether epidural anesthesia, given before 5 cm dilation, is associated with reduced uterine contractility[13] or an increase in cesareans for labor dystocia[14,15,16,17]. Epidurals are associated with a threefold increase in the use of oxytocin during labor, an increase in the length of the second stage, and an increase in instrumental deliveries[18]. In some large hospitals in the United States, epidurals are used by 80% or more of the women[13,19]. Trials of the effects of the timing of the administration of epidural analgesia would help maximize the safety and cost-effectiveness of this expensive procedure. Postponing medications in the first place may be a better choice if the woman can utilize non-pharmacological pain-coping measures.

## Dehydration

Dehydration may contribute to dystocia by decreasing contraction intensity and efficiency. Most women, if encouraged to drink as desired and if offered a beverage frequently, will avoid dehydration. The restriction of all oral fluids for healthy women in normal labor is rare, although limiting the amounts and choice of fluids (for example, sips or ice chips only, water only) is widespread[20,21], especially with caregivers who perceive all laboring women as pre-surgical patients. They prefer intravenous hydration, even though it carries its own set of potential risks and drawbacks (neonatal hypoglycemia, maternal and fetal hyponatremia, maternal psychological stress)[5]. One simple solution to preventing dehydration is to encourage the woman to drink to thirst (water or fruit juice), and noting whether and how much she is drinking.

Some women vomit frequently throughout labor, which increases the risk of dehydration. Contrary to widely held opinion, withholding oral fluids under such circumstances does not decrease the likelihood of vomiting, though it may decrease the volume. In fact, sips of water or juice may make the woman feel better, even if she continues to vomit, but she may require intravenous fluids for adequate hydration.

---

**Note regarding food and fluids in labor**

A policy of withholding food and fluids from laboring women became widespread in North America and the United Kingdom in the 1940s and 1950s and remained until the 1980s. The policy was based on concerns over the dangers of general anesthesia for laboring women who had food in their stomachs, because they were more likely to vomit and aspirate the vomitus (food particles and gastric acid) while under general anesthesia. Fasting has not been proven to solve such problems; in fact, the gastric secretions are actually more acidic and thus more damaging if aspirated than when one is not fasting. Safe anesthesia techniques appear to be the best safeguard against aspiration. Furthermore, the use of general anesthesia has been almost entirely replaced by epidural and spinal anesthesia (for cesareans). As a result, policies of 'nothing by mouth,' at least in early labor, have declined. In fact, the risks of withholding nourishment, especially during a long labor (ketosis, hypoglycemia, maternal hunger and thirst), may be greater than the risks of general anesthesia for the low risk woman. Digestion usually slows down by active labor and the woman has little appetite for food, though she will probably want to continue to drink fluids.

---

**4**

## WHEN THE CAUSE OF INADEQUATE CONTRACTIONS IS UNKNOWN

(See Chapter 2, page 25, 'Techniques to elicit stronger contractions'). The following measures may lead to stronger contractions:

- Nipple stimulation: Most trials of nipple stimulation have investigated its usefulness as an alternative to oxytocin in contraction stress testing (a test which has been determined to be 'likely to be ineffective or harmful'[22]) and its effectiveness in ripening the cervix or inducing labor. Midwives, however, especially in out-of-hospital settings, sometimes try having the woman or her partner lightly stroke one or both nipples to increase oxytocin release and augment contractions. Contractions and fetal well-being should be monitored for the possibility that the resulting contractions may be excessive or that fetal well-being will be compromised. Tetanic contractions with nipple stimulation have been reported in high risk women (with indications for induction) in late pregnancy. There has been little study of nipple stimulation in healthy women to augment labor contractions[23].

- Walking improves effectiveness of contractions[11].

- Acupressure may be used to stimulate more frequent contractions. Acupressure has never been scientifically evaluated for effectiveness or safety, although no harmful effects have been reported when used properly. See Chapter 7, page 174, for instructions.

- Bathing during the active phase of labor may enhance contractions if stress, tension, or anxiety is a contributing factor. The relaxation and pain relief resulting from immersion in water may result in improved progress. Timing of the bath may be important. As stated in Chapter 3, using the bath in early labor may slow the contractions, whereas using it in the active phase often speeds dilation[24].

In summary, contractions may be slowed or weakened by policies that restrict movement, withhold food or drink, raise maternal anxiety, overmedicate the woman, or medicate her too early in labor. A policy of prevention by avoiding such policies seems desirable, since the effects are difficult to reverse with physiological interventions. If the above measures fail to improve the effectiveness of contractions, then artificial rupture of the membranes and intravenous oxytocin may become necessary.

# IF THERE IS A PERSISTENT CERVICAL LIP OR A SWOLLEN CERVIX

Position changes can often be used to reduce a persistent cervical lip or (that is, a cervix that is fully dilated except for an anterior lip) alleviate a swollen cervix, which may become increasingly edematous. Sometimes the lip is formed by uneven pressure by the presenting part on the cervix. The following approaches may correct the problem.

## Position changes

Often the woman seems to know what to do, and in seeking comfort, also places herself in a position favorable for reducing the anterior lip. If that does not succeed, time and positions that reduce the pressure on the cervix seem to be the best positions to use. Gravity-neutral or anti-gravity positions, such as hands and knees, kneeling on a ball or the open knee–chest position (Figs 4.37–4.39) may move the fetal head away from the cervix and take some of the pressure off. Sidelying, semi-prone, or standing positions (Figs 4.40–4.42) redistribute the pressure on the cervix and may reduce the lip.

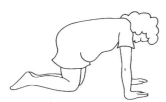

**Fig. 4.37**   Hands and knees.

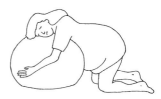

**Fig. 4.38**   Kneeling with a ball.

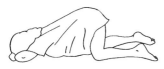

**Fig. 4.39**   Open knee–chest position.

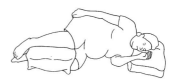

**Fig. 4.40**   Lateral.

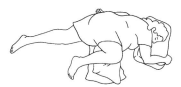

**Fig. 4.41** Semi-prone with lower arm back.

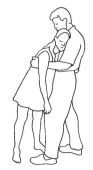

**Fig. 4.42** Standing, leaning on partner.

## Other methods

Immersion in a bath of deep water: the 'weightlessness' and buoyancy reduce the effects of gravity and may relieve pressure on the cervix.

(We are intrigued by a suggestion in a midwifery text for reducing swelling in the cervix: the application of crushed ice, placed in the finger of a sterile glove and applied to the cervix[25]. We have no experience and no published studies of this technique.)

---

*Note on asynclitism and the occiput posterior (OP) position:*

Asymmetrical dilation (and the formation of a cervical lip) often occurs when the fetus is asynclitic or OP. See pages 54–9, for positions that may resolve these malpositions.

---

## Manual reduction of a cervical lip

Sometimes a more aggressive approach to an anterior lip with a cervix that is almost completely dilated may be warranted: manual reduction[26]. This painful procedure should be fully explained to the woman, along with the expected benefit of shortening the time until complete dilation. If she agrees, then the caregiver, between contractions, presses the cervix back over the fetal head and above the pubic arch. The caregiver holds the cervix in that position through the next contraction. The woman pushes through the contraction in hopes of moving the fetus down below the pubic arch, thus preventing the anterior lip from re-forming.

## IF EMOTIONAL DYSTOCIA IS SUSPECTED

The term 'emotional dystocia' refers to dysfunctional labor caused by emotional distress and the resulting excessive production of catecholamines. High catecholamine levels reduce the circulation to the uterus and placenta during labor, and cause inefficient contractions and reduced fetal oxygenation. In addition, constant disturbance in a busy, strange environment may cause the woman to be unable to 'turn off' her neo-cortex and labor instinctually. See page 12 for the biological basis of emotional dystocia.

### Indicators of emotional dystocia

A woman experiencing emotional dystocia may:

- express or display fear or anxiety
- ask many questions, or remain very alert to her surroundings
- exhibit very 'needy' behavior
- display extreme modesty
- exhibit strong reactions to mild contractions or to examinations
- show a high degree of muscle tension
- appear demanding, distrustful, angry, or resentful toward staff
- exhibit a strong need for control over caregivers' actions
- seem 'out of control' in labor (in extreme pain, writhing, panicked, screaming, unresponsive to helpful suggestions or questions)
- seem very controlled in her responses to contractions, but express fear that she will lose control as labor becomes more intense
- or may not exhibit any behaviors that would lead one to consider emotional dystocia. (See Chapter 3, page 35 and Chapter 7, pages 179–82, for ways to discover if fear or anxiety may be contributing to the dystocia.)

### Predisposing factors for emotional dystocia

Whatever the woman's fears or anxieties are, she probably cannot simply 'snap out of it.' Her emotional state results partly from pre-existing factors which may include:

- previous difficult births
- previous traumatic hospitalizations
- childhood abuse: physical, sexual, or emotional (see page 75 on the impact of sexual abuse on childbearing women)
- dysfunctional family of origin (mental illness, substance abuse, fighting by parents, or other family problems)
- fears about current serious health problems
- domestic violence (previous or present)
- cultural factors, including beliefs leading to extreme shame when viewed nude, or when viewed in labor by men
- language barrier, or inability to hear or understand what is happening or what is being done
- substance abuse by the woman
- death of her own mother (especially in childbirth or at a young age)
- beliefs resulting from what she has been told about labor (for example, the woman whose sibling was handicapped by a 'birth injury', or whose mother had a 'terrible time' giving birth to her).

## Helping the woman state her fears

**4**

Of course, maternity professionals are not expected to provide psychotherapy. On the other hand, addressing her concerns by asking a few sensitive questions between contractions may help the woman state her fears and allow those around her to give more effective care: 'What was going through your mind during that contraction?', or 'How are you feeling right now?', or 'Do you have any idea why your labor is slowing down?'. She may indicate any of the following common fears or others, which could interfere with labor progress:

- dread of increasing pain
- fear of damage or disfigurement to her own body, including stretching, episiotomy, tears, stitching, or a cesarean, and 'never being the same again'
- fear of uterine rupture, if she has had a cesarean before
- fear that labor will harm her baby (a belief that a cesarean is safer and easier for the baby)
- fear of loss of control, of modesty, or of dignity; 'acting like a fool' or 'losing face' (shame)

- fear of invasive procedures, such as vaginal exams, injections, blood tests or others
- fear of strangers, the caregivers who have power and authority over her
- fear of being unable to care for her baby adequately, of being a 'terrible mother'
- fear of abandonment by the baby's father, her caregiver, or others
- fear of dying (Note: a brief transient period of fear of dying in the late first stage, associated with a surge of catecholamines and the 'fetal ejection reflex' (see page 12) is not unusual, and it is not associated with dystocia[27]. A deep prolonged persistent fear throughout pregnancy and labor is what we are referring to here.)

It is important to state that most women have some fear or anxiety about labor, birth, and the impact of a new child on their lives. This does not mean that all those women will have labor dystocia. For some women, however, emotional issues are powerful enough to interfere with an efficient labor pattern. Being able to detect those women and help them may reduce the negative impact of emotional distress. In any case, your sensitivity and attentiveness will contribute to a woman's sense of being cared for and cared about.

After having identified (or, having guessed) the woman's fears, it may be helpful to do some or all of the following:

- Provide language interpreters and culturally competent or culturally sensitive caregivers, if needed.

- Restate what she has said to check that you understand ('It sounds as if you're afraid of what the labor might do to your baby. Is that right?'). If the woman confirms this, then:

- Validate her fear, rather than dismissing it. 'Yes, other women have told me they worried about that too,' or 'That must be frightening. We're also concerned about babies during labor and that's why we check your baby's heartbeat frequently.'

- Provide reassuring information (but not empty promises). 'Listening to his heartbeat, he sounds just fine right now. Would you like to know how babies adapt to contractions during labor? They have some really amazing coping mechanisms. . .'

- Observe her affect and behavior during conversations and elicit further concerns or needs.

- Between contractions let her know that, after the baby is born, there are helpful resources available to her (and follow up with this information later). For example, if the woman is worried about being an inadequate mother, she might be relieved to know there are parenting classes and support groups, and a hotline she can call for help at any time, day or night. Helping her recognize that labor is not the time to address her fears about parenthood, while also reassuring her that she will not be alone with her concerns, may ease her anxiety enough that labor progress will resume. Perhaps calming her conscious fears will help her enter a more relaxed state in which the 'primitive' parts of her brain will dominate and promote the labor process.

- Provide ideas (non-judgmentally) that the woman can use to alter the situation. If the woman feels 'helpless' lying down, she might feel strong and active standing up.

- Visualization and reframing can be powerful tools to help a woman overcome her fear. For example, if she expresses concern about her 'poor baby's head being forced through that tiny tight opening', she can be helped to imagine her 'little baby *nuzzling* his head down in that *soft stretchy place*' (describing her ripe cervix and vagina as being as soft and stretchy as the inside of her cheek when she presses inside it with her tongue).

- If the woman is unable to cope with overwhelming physical sensations, she may benefit from massage, hydrotherapy, or pain medication.

Chart 4.4 summarizes ways to help women when emotional distress is a likely cause of dystocia. See page 75 for the special needs of childhood abuse survivors.

## How to help a woman for whom emotional distress is a likely cause of labor dystocia

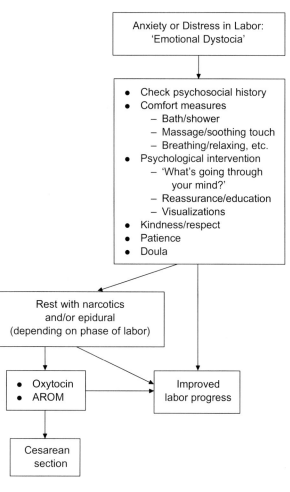

**Chart 4.4**

## Special needs of childhood abuse survivors

A woman who was sexually or physically abused as a child may have great anxieties in labor, especially related to:

- invasive procedures: vaginal exams, other instruments placed in the vagina, blood tests, or I-Vs that remind her of the abuse
- lack of control: as a child she was hurt when she was out of control and vulnerable. She may have learned never to lose control
- modesty, nakedness, exposure issues
- powerful authority figures (midwives, nurses, doctors) who know more than she, and who do painful things to her: as a child she was a victim of those with authority over her
- being asked to 'relax, surrender, or yield to the contractions' with the promise that it won't hurt so much: she may have been told similar things during the abuse
- pushing her baby out of her vagina: the prospect of pain and damage may remind her of sexual abuse.

Sometimes an abuse survivor seems difficult or demanding when she responds very emotionally or angrily to the above items. It is important that the caregiver does not take her reaction personally and keeps in mind that she has very good reason to react the way she does, but also that the caregiver is not the reason. If a caregiver observes some of the behaviors listed above, she or he should suspect a history of abuse, and try to be patient and kind, and to accommodate to her special needs even if they seem unusual or unreasonable. If she feels emotionally safe, her labor may progress more normally, and she may reap other psychological benefits as well.

## INCOMPATIBILITY OR POOR RELATIONSHIP WITH STAFF

If the woman has developed a poor relationship with any staff member, it will help to discuss the specific concerns or differences of opinion with the staff member him- or herself, or with that person's superior. Sometimes all the woman needs is to be listened to, respected, and taken seriously; then she may be more able to trust the people around her. Perhaps the staff will be able to make some compromises in their usual routines in order to meet her needs, while still accomplishing those clinical tasks that are essential to basic safety.

Sometimes the simplest solution, once the woman discovers that she and her assigned nurse or midwife are incompatible, is to change to someone else to provide a fresh start in the relationship. There is no need to lay blame, only to recognize the incompatibility and to do something about it. (Note: This is less likely to be a problem where a policy of 'continuity of caregiver' is in place, as it is in some parts of the UK.)

If it is possible to anticipate these difficulties before labor, it makes sense to suggest that this patient be assigned to a particularly diplomatic or understanding midwife or nurse, and that the woman bring a doula (professional labor support person) with her in labor. The doula can provide extra psychological support to relieve the burden on the caregiver. It also helps if staff can be flexible to a woman's unusual requests and be willing to meet them, if possible.

## IF THE SOURCE OF THE WOMAN'S ANXIETY CANNOT BE IDENTIFIED

**4**

Sometimes a caregiver cannot understand why the labor is not going well. All the physical factors seem normal, and the woman does not exhibit any particular psychosocial problems. It sometimes helps to wait until after a contraction and ask her, 'Could you tell me what was going through your mind during that contraction?'. If necessary, ask, 'Anything else?'. The answer she gives may be a clue to her emotional state. For example, if she responds, 'I am just trying to do the breathing and relaxation I learned in childbirth class,' it is clear that she is coping, and should be encouraged to continue the self-comforting measures. If, however, she says she is afraid, or feels helpless, or it hurts terribly, or she cannot do it much longer, she is obviously in distress, and the caregiver can help (in culturally appropriate ways) by acknowledging her distress, reassuring her, addressing her fear, holding her hand, and helping her and her partner with some self-comforting measures. (See Chapter 2.) One notable study found that women who expressed distress in early labor were more likely to have longer labors, more fetal distress, and all the interventions that go along with these problems[28]. If emotional distress can be identified and alleviated early in labor, these damaging effects of distress may be prevented with extra support, reassurance, encouragement, and assistance.

# CONCLUSION

The psycho-emotional factors that influence labor progress are less well understood than the physical factors, but they may be as important. Try to remain sensitive to this aspect of childbirth. Your influence on the mind–body connection in labor may be greater than you think.

# REFERENCES

1. O'Driscoll, K., Meagher, D. and Boylan, P. (1993) *Active Management of Labour*. Mosby Year Book Europe, London.
2. Friedman, E.A. (1995) Dystocia and 'failure to progress' in labor. In: *Cesarean Section: Guidelines for Appropriate Utilization*, Flamm, B.L. and Quilligan, E.J. (eds). Springer-Verlag, New York.
3. Crowther, C., Enkin, M., Keirse, M.J.N.C. and Brown, I. (1989) Monitoring the progress of labour. In: *Effective Care in Pregnancy and Childbirth*, vol. 2, Chalmers, I., Enkin, M. and Keirse, M.J.N.C. (eds). Oxford University Press, Oxford.
4. Sweet, B. and Tiran, D. (eds) (1997) *Mayes' Midwifery: A Textbook for Midwives*, 12th edition. Baillière Tindall, London.
5. Enkin, M., Keirse, M.J.N.C., Renfrew, M. and Neilsen, J. (1995) Monitoring progress of labour. In: *A Guide to Effective Care in Pregnancy and Childbirth* (2nd edition). Oxford University Press, Oxford.
6. Keirse, M.J.N.C. (1989) Augmentation of labour. In: *Effective Care in Pregnancy and Childbirth*, vol. 2, Chalmers, I., Enkin, M. and Keirse, M.J.N.C. (eds). Oxford University Press, Oxford.
7. Butler, J., Abrams, B., Parker, J., Roberts, J. and Laros, R. (1993) Supportive nurse–midwife care is associated with a reduced incidence of cesarean section. *Am. J. Obstet. Gynecol.* **168**, 1407–13.
8. King, J.M. (1993) *Back Labor No More!! What Every Woman Should Know Before Labor*. Plenary Systems, Dallas.
9. Sutton, J. and Scott, P. (1996) *Understanding and Teaching Optimal Foetal Positioning*. Birth Concepts, Tauranga, NZ.
10. Fenwick, L. and Simkin, P. (1987) Maternal positioning to prevent or alleviate dystocia. *Clin. Obstet. Gynecol.* **30 (1)**, 83–9.
11. Roberts, J. (1989) Maternal position during the first stage of labour. In: *Effective Care in Pregnancy and Childbirth*, vol. 2, Chalmers, I., Enkin, M. and Keirse, M.J.N.C. (eds). Oxford University Press, Oxford.
12. Bloom, S.L., McIntire, D.D., Kelly, M.A., Beimer, H.L., Burpo, R.H., Garcia, M.A. and Leveno, K.J. (1998) Lack of effect of walking on labor and delivery. *N. Engl. J. Med.* **339**, 76–9.
13. Newton, E.R., Schroeder, B.C., Knape, K.G. and Bennett, B.L. (1995) Epidural analgesia and uterine function. *Obstet. Gynecol.* **85 (5) Part 1**, 749–55.

**4**

14. Thorp, J.A., Hu, D.H., Albin, R.M., McNill, J., Meyer, B.A., Gohen, G.R. and Yeast, J.D. (1993) The effect of intrapartum epidural analgesia on nulliparous labor: A randomized, controlled, prospective trial. *Am. J. Obstet. Gynecol.* **169 (4)**, 851–8.

15. Ramin, S.M., Gambling, D.R., Lucas, M.J., Sharma, S.K., Disawi, J.E. and Leveno, K.J. (1995) Randomized trial of epidural versus intravenous analgesia during labor. *Obstet. Gynecol.* **86 (5)**, 783–9.

16. Chestnut, D.H., McGrath, J.M. and Vincent, R.D. (1994) Does early administration of epidural analgesia affect obstetric outcome in nulliparous women who are in spontaneous labor? *Anesthesiology* **80 (6)**, 1201–8.

17. Chestnut, D.H., Vincent, R.D. and McGrath, J.M. (1994) Does early administration of epidural analgesia affect obstetric outcome in nulliparous women who are receiving intravenous oxytocin? *Anesthesiology* **80 (6)**, 1193–1200.

18. MIDIRS and The NHS Centre for Reviews and Dissemination (1997) Epidural pain relief during labour. In the Informed Choice for Professionals Series.

19. Whalley, J. (1998) *Survey of Hospitals and Alternative Birth Services.* Childbirth Education Association of Seattle, Seattle.

20. Berry, H. (1997) Feast or famine? Oral intake during labour: current evidence and practice. *Br. J. Midwif.* **5 (7)**, 413–17.

21. Sharp, D.A. (1997) Restriction of oral intake for women in labour. *Br. J. Midwif.* **5 (7)**, 408–12.

22. Enkin, M., Keirse, M.J.N.C., Renfrew, M. and Neilsen, J. (1995) Table 6 (p. 410). In: *A Guide to Effective Care in Pregnancy and Childbirth*, 2nd edition. Oxford University Press, Oxford.

23. Stein, J.L., Bardeguez, A.D., Verma, U. and Tegani, N. (1990) Nipple stimulation for labor augmentation. *J. Reprod. Med.* **35 (7)**, 710–14.

24. Eriksson, M., Mattson, L.A. and Ladfors, L. (1997) Early or late bath during the first stage of labour: A randomised study of 200 women. *Midwifery* **13**, 146–8.

25. Davis, E. (1997) *Heart and Hands: A Midwife's Guide to Pregnancy and Birth*, 3rd edition. Celestial Arts, Berkeley.

26. Varney, H. (1997) *Varney's Midwifery*, 3rd edition. Jones & Bartlett, Boston.

27. Odent, M. (1992) *The Nature of Birth and Breastfeeding.* Bergin & Garvey, Westport, CT.

28. Wuitchik, M., Bakal, D. and Lipshitz, J. (1989) The clinical significance of pain and cognitive activity in latent labor. *Obstet. Gynecol.* **73 (1)**, 35–41.

**4**

# Chapter 5

# Prolonged Second Stage of Labor

5

## DEFINITIONS OF THE SECOND STAGE

By definition, the second stage of labor begins with complete dilation of the cervix and ends with the birth of the baby. The clinical significance of complete dilation is controversial. In North America the usual conduct of the second stage is based on a desire for a speedy delivery, and calls for the woman to commence maximal breath-holding and bearing-down efforts when she is discovered to be fully dilated, even though her urge to push may occur before or after complete dilation. If the urge to push occurs before complete dilation, the woman is told to resist pushing by panting throughout each contraction (see page 61, for further discussion of what to do with a premature urge to push). If the urge to push is not present when she is completely dilated, the desire for a speedy delivery leads the caregiver to exhort the woman to begin pushing.

In the UK, however, being completely dilated is not believed to be as important as it is in North America. Rather, the conduct of second stage is based on the onset of the 'expulsive phase,' that is, the time when the woman first exhibits involuntary expulsive efforts (an urge to push). This approach seems to have a basis in physiology since, in the normal course of events, contractions sometimes diminish temporarily around the time of full dilation.

## THE PHASES OF THE SECOND STAGE

The second stage of labor can be divided into phases (the latent phase and the active phase), just as the first stage is. Each phase represents different behaviors of the woman, and different physiological accomplishments.

### The latent phase of the second stage

A lull in uterine activity around the time of complete dilation is frequently observed and is sometimes referred to as the 'latent phase of the second stage'[1], the 'resting phase'[2], or the 'rest and be thankful phase'[3].

Although a latent phase in the second stage is often perceived as abnormal and may be treated as uterine inertia, it is probably a physiological phenomenon relating to the retraction of the cervix around the head and the descent of the fetal head into the vaginal canal[4,5]. E.A. Friedman refers to this as the 'deceleration phase' of the first stage (the last 1 or 2 cm of dilation), during which the maximum rate of descent usually begins. The following hypothesis may help to explain the frequently observed lull in uterine activity in the early second stage[1] (Fig. 5.1).

- During most of the first stage of labor the uterus is tightly wrapped around the fetus. Uterine contractions in the first stage not only dilate the cervix, but also shorten the uterine muscle fibers, which gradually reduce the intrauterine space and presses the fetus down.

- The last 2 cm of dilation are accompanied by cervical retraction

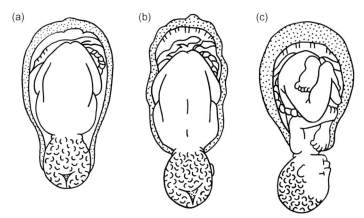

**Fig. 5.1** Latent phase of second stage. Fetal head slips through cervix, and uterine muscle slackens. Uterine muscle fibres shorten until the uterus is once again tightly wrapped around fetal trunk. (a) Fetus in uterus at full dilation. (b) Head out of uterus, which slackens. (c) Uterus shortened and thickened around fetal torso.

around the head (or presenting part), and the beginnings of descent of the head into the vaginal canal[4].

- The fetal head represents 25–30% of its entire body. When the head (representing one-quarter of the contents of the uterus) slips through the cervix, the uterine muscle may slacken as it is no longer tightly stretched around the fetal trunk. It must now 'catch up' with the fetus.

- This 'catching up' consists of shortening of the uterine muscle fibers (as happened gradually in the first stage), further reducing the intrauterine space until once again the uterine muscle is tightly wrapped around the fetal trunk. This may take minutes or longer, during which contractions are weak or unnoticeable, and the woman may doze. Fetal position and station are two of the factors that determine whether and when the woman will experience a resting phase, and also how long it lasts.

- The contractions resume and the woman experiences an increasingly powerful urge to push, accompanied by a documented spurt in oxytocin release[6,7].

This hypothesis is consistent with our knowledge of uterine physiology in labor, with Friedman's classic observations of normal labor progress, and with the numerous observational studies of maternal spontaneous bearing-down efforts that document an increasing urge to push and greater spontaneous bearing-down efforts with time and descent of the presenting part[8,9].

### Asking women to push during the latent phase of the second stage

In the absence of contractions the fetal heart tones usually remain reassuring. With no interventions at all, the contractions usually resume within 5–30 minutes. During the latent phase, the woman gets some rest, her spirits rise, and she begins to look forward to delivering her child.

In North America, caregivers sometimes misinterpret the latent phase to mean labor has slowed down, and make efforts to speed the second stage, by

- enlisting the woman's maximal expulsive efforts, which are exhausting and non-productive; or by
- ordering oxytocin (Pitocin) to augment uterine contractions. Though widely used to augment labor, oxytocin is not free from potential adverse effects, such as tetanic contractions and fetal distress[10].

These unnecessary interventions are less likely to be used when the British approach is used. 'In uncomplicated labour, the timing of the decision to encourage maternal effort is usually when the presenting part is "on view" or there is obvious descent of the presenting part with an uncontrollable urge to push'[11].

### What if the latent phase of the second stage persists?

If the lull in uterine activity persists for more than 20 or 30 minutes, the caregiver may continue monitoring and waiting, or may, if the woman agrees, initiate measures to bring on contractions and an urge to push. These measures may include a change in the woman's position to sitting upright (in bed or on the toilet), squatting, or walking; 'trial' expulsive efforts (breath-holding and bearing down) by the woman; acupressure; and nipple stimulation. See the Toolkit in Chapter 7 and pages 25, 67 for specific descriptions and precautions regarding these measures.

Many professionals now await evidence of an urge to push before checking the woman's cervix. By doing so, they are less likely to perceive second stage as prolonged. They prefer the two-fold definition of second stage: complete dilation plus spontaneous expulsive efforts.

## The active phase of the second stage

The active phase of the second stage is characterized by an involuntary urge to push and descent of the fetus. It is sometimes referred to as the 'pelvic division' of labor[3], the 'press period'[12], or the descent phase[1]. The woman's contractions, her expulsive efforts, and her body positions are the forces that combine to deliver her child. Recent research regarding expulsive efforts (positions, breathing, bearing down) for second stage has resulted in some new thinking about how women should push and the role of clinical personnel in assisting the woman at this time.

### *Directed expulsive efforts*

Just how a woman should 'push' is the subject of some disagreement among caregivers. Until recently, the usual expectation has been that the woman should lie flat on her back or in a semi-reclining position; draw her legs up toward her shoulders; and when the contraction begins, she takes a deep breath, holds it, and strains (bears down) maximally for at least 10 seconds; releases her breath; quickly takes another; and repeats this routine until the contraction ends. The caregiver actively, enthusiastically, and sometimes loudly directs these efforts.

This technique of maximal maternal effort was devised by natural childbirth advocates in the 1950s as a way to overcome the anti-gravity effects of the mandatory lithotomy position, and to deliver the baby quickly enough to avoid forceps. It was incorporated into nursing and midwifery practice and remains the custom today[13]. There are problems with this approach, however.

### *Physiological effects of prolonged breath-holding and straining on the woman*

Prolonged breath-holding and straining lead to (Chart 5.1):

- a closed pressure system in her chest, which leads to decreases in venous return, cardiac output, and maternal arterial blood pressure
- an increase in the peripheral stasis of blood in her head, face, arms, and legs. Her face reddens and if an intravenous line is in place, blood often backs up in the I-V catheter
- a decrease in maternal blood oxygen levels and blood flow to the placenta
- an increase in maternal carbon dioxide levels until she gasps for air
- a sudden increase in her blood pressure as she gasps for air, causing bursting of tiny blood vessels in the whites of her eyes, her face, neck, and eyes (petechial hemorrhages)
- rapid distension of the vaginal canal and pelvic musculature, along with stretching of supportive ligaments, leading to perineal trauma and possible urinary stress incontinence
- maternal exhaustion.

*These effects are well tolerated by young healthy women, but may present risks for older or some high-risk women, especially if such efforts are required for several hours.*

**5**

---

MATERNAL EFFECTS:

Prolonged breath-holding and straining (Valsalva maneuver)

$\rightarrow$ a closed pressure system in chest, $\rightarrow$ $\downarrow$ venous return, $\downarrow$ cardiac output, $\downarrow$ blood pressure, and $\downarrow$ blood flow to placenta.

Also $\uparrow$ in peripheral stasis of blood (head and face, arms and legs) $\rightarrow$ red face.

Mother's $O_2$ levels $\downarrow$, and $CO_2$ levels $\uparrow$, $\rightarrow$ gasping for air, $\rightarrow$ sudden $\uparrow$ in blood pressure, $\rightarrow$ capillaries in face, neck, and eyes bursting (petechial hemorrhages).

FETAL EFFECTS:

$\downarrow$ $O_2$ content in arterial blood and $\downarrow$ blood flow to placenta $\rightarrow$ $\downarrow$ $O_2$ available to fetus (fetal hypoxia).

---

**Chart 5.1**   The prolonged Valsalva maneuver (breath-holding and straining).

### Physiological effects of prolonged breath-holding and straining on the fetus

Fetal bradycardias sometimes occur when the woman holds her breath for prolonged periods and her straining may increase fetal head compression. If such bearing-down efforts are combined with a dorsal position, supine hypotension may exacerbate the bradycardia.

The decreases in maternal blood pressure, blood oxygen content, and placental blood flow cause a decrease in the oxygen available to the fetus (fetal hypoxia and acidosis)[9]. See Chart 5.1 for a summary of the effects of prolonged breath-holding and straining.

*These effects are well tolerated by a healthy, well nourished term fetus, but may distress the fetus who is pre-term, small for gestational age, already compromised earlier in labor, or is experiencing cord compression.*

Furthermore, such a bearing-down technique, while it may slightly shorten the second stage when compared with spontaneous bearing-down efforts in physiologically favorable positions, is not associated with better neonatal outcomes[9,14].

### Spontaneous expulsive efforts

Observational studies of women's behavior in the second stage reveal that women who have not been instructed on how to push breathe more and bear down less during second stage contractions than women who are told to use the prolonged maximal bearing-down efforts described above[8,9]. Also they change positions more[9,15]. With spontaneous bearing down in various positions, the undesirable side-effects of both prolonged maximal breath-holding and the supine position do not occur.

If a woman is not required to push in a prescribed manner or in a prescribed position, she may use a number of positions (sidelying, semi-reclining, standing, a supported squat, hands and knees, kneeling on both knees or with one knee elevated, squatting). She may hold her breath, moan, or even bellow during the contractions[16].

Most women experience an involuntary urge to push that comes and goes several times during each contraction. The woman's spontaneous bearing-down efforts last approximately 5–7 seconds, and she takes several breaths between bearing-down efforts[1,8,9,12,17].

As the second stage progresses and the fetus descends, the woman's spontaneous bearing-down efforts usually become more forceful and more frequent[8].

**5**

The caregiver's role is different when the woman is pushing spontaneously in physiological positions than when she is expected to push maximally in a supine position. The caregiver encourages and praises the woman's efforts and reassures her that the sensations she feels are normal. The caregiver emphasizes the value of relaxing her perineum rather than holding her breath or pushing to a count of 10. Chart 5.2 illustrates the caregiver's step-by-step approach to bearing-down (pushing) efforts once dilation is complete.

### *Diffuse pushing*

Sometimes the woman's spontaneous pushing is unfocused, or 'diffuse,' and results in little progress (Chart 5.3). It is almost as if all her

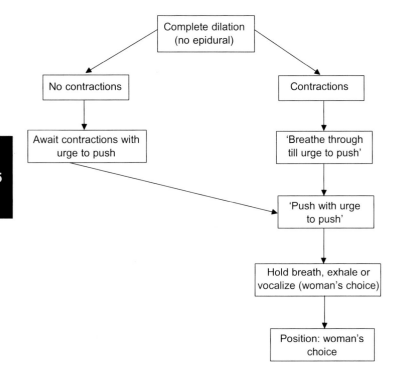

**Chart 5.2**   Spontaneous bearing down.

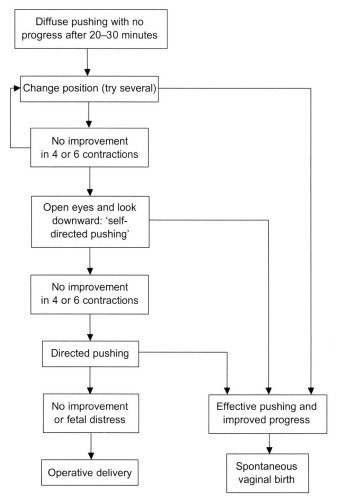

**Chart 5.3**

effort has no single direction. Such diffuse pushing seems to occur when the woman's eyes are tightly closed, and/or she is vocalizing continuously and there is little or no apparent progress after 20 or 30 minutes. The caregiver should first encourage the woman to change positions (see Toolkit, Chapter 6, for positions for second stage) – perhaps to a gravity-enhancing position. This often helps her to focus and push more effectively. If not, the caregiver should instruct the woman to open her eyes and direct her gaze (and her bearing-down efforts) toward her vagina, and think about pressing the baby out. The woman may need frequent reminders to keep her eyes open. It may also help to remind her of her baby, that her baby is bringing her pain out of her body. We call this 'self-directed pushing,' because the caregiver is helping the woman to direct her own bearing-down efforts.

These simple measures, opening her eyes and focusing on her baby, usually result in progress without fetal distress or serious perineal damage. In those rare cases when these measures do not succeed, the caregiver may need to resort to encouraging her to do the prolonged breath-holding and maximal bearing down described earlier. If so, one should remember that the fetus usually tolerates the second stage better when the woman holds her breath and strains for less than 7 seconds at a time[9,14,17].

### If the woman has an epidural

Though epidural analgesia confers excellent pain relief most of the time, there are tradeoffs involved which may increase the length of the second stage and increase the need for instrumental delivery[18,19]. The search for the safest and most effective management of the second stage with an epidural is a subject of great interest for caregivers as well as for childbearing women, especially in areas where epidural use is extremely prevalent. Certainly, epidurals change the second stage for both the woman and her caregivers (Chart 5.4). Consider the following:

- Normally, the woman's pelvic floor provides a resilient platform on which the fetal head can rotate, and the muscles lining the pelvis also provide a resilient cushion that encourages rotation. Pressure on these muscles elicits a stretch response that plays an important role in the cardinal movements of descent (flexion, internal rotation, extension, and external rotation). However, when anesthetized, there is a reduction in the tone of these muscles, which tends to inhibit rotation of the fetal head[19]. When combined with maximal breath-holding and straining by the woman, the likelihood of persistent malposition or a deep transverse arrest is greatly increased[20].

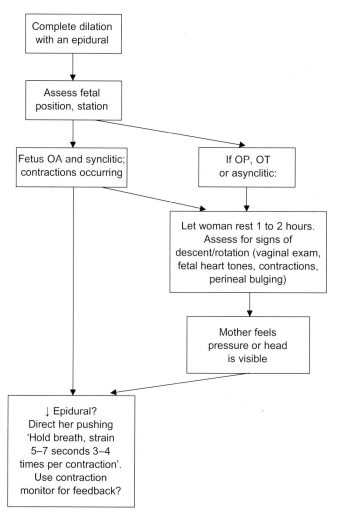

**Chart 5.4** Delayed pushing with an epidural.

- With anesthesia, the woman also lacks kinesthetic feedback to help her discover how to push effectively.

- An anesthetized woman is restricted to the few positions that she can assume without full sensation or use of her legs. These are usually limited to sidelying, supine, semi-sitting, sitting upright, or – in some cases with light anesthesia and good physical support – squatting and hands and knees. Changing position usually requires assistance.

- Anesthesia may interfere with the usual spurt of endogenous oxytocin that is associated with pressure of the presenting part within the lower vagina[6]. Normally the pressure on the posterior vaginal wall or the pelvic floor signals the pituitary gland to release more oxytocin, resulting in stronger contractions, a greater urge to push, and more pressure on the pelvic floor. Anesthesia blocks this oxytocin-producing feedback loop, and progress is often impaired.

- Because of the reduced urge to push with an epidural, pushing requires a greater voluntary effort than pushing in response to an urge.

Some of the above problems may be partly remedied by the following approaches to epidural management:

- Using lower concentrations of the anesthetic when the epidural is first placed, possibly combining it with low dose narcotics, may allow more awareness and more motor control.

- Discontinuing or decreasing the dose of the epidural at the end of the first stage of labor may allow the return of sensation and an urge to push. It may also improve pelvic muscle tone, thus encouraging rotation. The resulting return of pain for the woman may be unacceptable, however.

- Delaying pushing for up to two hours, or until the fetal head is OA[19] or becomes visible at the vaginal outlet (when the labia are parted) may reduce the need for forceps rotation without risk to the newborn[20,21]. By delaying pushing and avoiding forcing descent, the malpositioned fetus will often in time rotate and align well in the pelvis. Once OA, directed pushing is most appropriate[22].

*Note:* A recent randomized controlled trial[23] comparing early versus late pushing in women with epidural analgesia found no difference in length of second stage between the two groups. There was, however, no analysis of the subgroup of women with unrotated or asynclitic fetuses. Without data on this group, it may make more sense to delay pushing until the head is OA, synclitic, and/or visible at the introitus.

- Removing the time limit for second stage with an epidural improves the chances of a spontaneous delivery without risk to the neonate. Even if rotation and descent are slow, as long as fetus and woman are tolerating it well, many caregivers see no medical reason to intervene.

- If the woman is unaware of an urge to push and an electronic fetal monitor is being used, the monitor can be used as a biofeedback device to encourage her bearing-down efforts once it is appropriate for her to push. By positioning the monitor within her view, she can be directed to watch the digital contraction indicator as she bears down. The increase in the numbers gives her feedback that her efforts are making a difference. The device can be used to give her incentive to push effectively ('Go for 90! That's it, 70, 73, 77, 84, 90! Great!').

- When the woman is to begin pushing, the caregiver may have to become quite directive, telling the woman when to breathe and when to bear down. Breath-holding for no more than 7 seconds at a time, with several breaths between, results in better fetal oxygenation than prolonged and constant breath-holding and straining.

If progress is slow, changing positions every 20 to 30 minutes often improves progress. Chart 5.4 summarizes the instructions for delayed pushing with an epidural.

## How long an active phase of second stage is too long?

Although it is standard practice for many doctors and midwives to limit the duration of second stage labor to two hours from complete dilation to birth, there is no scientific rationale for such an approach. The length of the second stage is not as important to a good outcome as the status of mother and baby *during* that time. Individual care and careful assessment often allow more time for second stage with no compromise in the well-being of mother or baby.

An extensive review of the scientific literature on this issue concludes, 'There is no evidence to suggest that, when the second stage of labour is progressing and the condition of both woman and fetus is satisfactory, the imposition of any upper arbitrary limit on its duration is justified. Such limits should be discarded[9]'. E.A. Friedman agrees: 'The recommendations for management of the prolonged second stage derived from the observations of no ill effect from long second stages include admonitions to avoid reflexively considering cesarean section when a patient's second stage extends beyond any arbitrary duration'[24].

## POSSIBLE ETIOLOGIES AND SOLUTIONS FOR SECOND-STAGE DYSTOCIA

The challenge for caregivers in a long second stage is to detect reasons for the slow progress and institute appropriate corrective measures. The choice of early interventions depends, to an extent, on the presumed etiology, although a trial and error approach is sometimes warranted.

### Positions and other strategies for suspected occiput posterior (OP) or persistent occiput transverse (OT) fetuses

Figures 5.2a, b, c, and d illustrate abdominal and vaginal views of the OP and OT positions.

As long as the woman is well supported and she has no musculoskeletal or medical problems, and her fetus is monitored, a wide variety of positions may be used to promote descent. Some of these make it quite difficult or inconvenient for the caregiver to conduct the delivery. Therefore, once it is clear that birth is imminent, the woman might be asked to move from one of these inconvenient positions, and assume a position in which the birth attendant is able to assist if necessary.

(a)

(b)

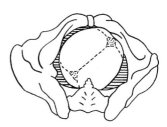

(c)

(d)

5

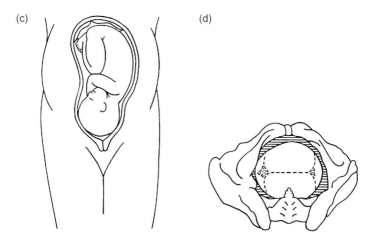

**Fig. 5.2**    (a) Right occiput posterior – abdominal view. (b) Right occiput posterior in synclitism – vaginal view. (c) Left occiput transverse – abdominal view. (d) Left occiput transverse – vaginal view.

### Why not the dorsal position?

Dorsal positions tend to exacerbate malpositions and deny the effects of gravity. See pages 59–60, 116–117 and Chapter 6 for information on the disadvantages of supine positions. In some specific situations, the advantages of exaggerated lithotomy may outweigh the risks. For most women, the positions shown in Figs 5.3–5.21 are more effective in promoting fetal rotation and descent, and may be more comfortable for the woman than the dorsal positions. Changing positions every 20 minutes when progress is slow may help solve the problem. Even if the fetus cannot be rotated, these same measures may make a vaginal birth possible in a persistent OP or OT position.

### Leaning forward while kneeling, standing, or sitting

These positions (Figs 5.3–5.7) take advantage of gravity to encourage rotation of the fetal trunk from posterior to anterior. Back pain, common with OP, is also relieved because the pressure of the fetal head on the sacrum is relieved. See the Toolkit, Chapter 6 for more information.

(a)   (b)

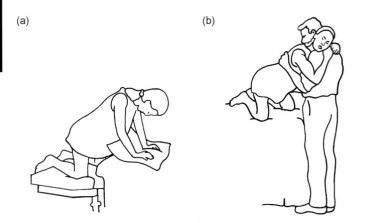

**Fig. 5.3**   (a) Kneeling on foot of bed. (b) Kneeling, leaning on partner to push.

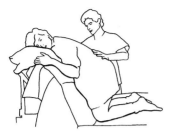

**Fig. 5.4** Kneeling, leaning on the raised head of the bed.

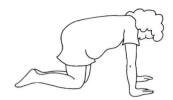

**Fig. 5.5** Hands and knees.

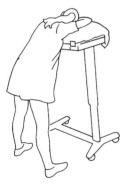

**Fig. 5.6** Standing, leaning on a tray table.

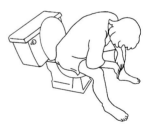

**Fig. 5.7** Sitting forward on toilet.

**5**

### *Squatting positions*

These utilize weight-bearing with hip abduction to widen the pelvic outlet, which may enlarge the space in the pelvic basin enough to promote rotation and descent. See Figs 5.8 and 5.9, and, for more information on squatting Chapter 6, pages 143–8.

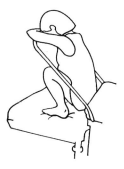

**Fig. 5.8** Squatting with bar.

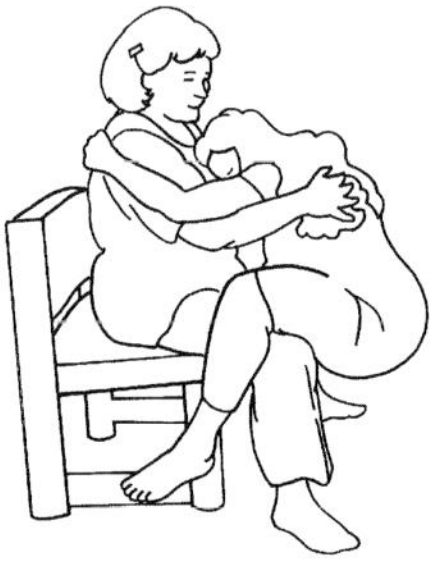

**Fig. 5.9** Lap squatting.

### *Asymmetrical positions*

In these each of the woman's legs is in a different position (for example, one knee up and one knee down). This changes the shape of the pelvis in ways that are different from 'symmetrical' positions such as squatting, and hands and knees. The pelvic joints on one side of the pelvis widen more than the joints on the other side. Sometimes the fetus is more likely to rotate with such positions. See Figs 5.10–5.12, and pages 58 and 141–3 for more information on asymmetrical positions.

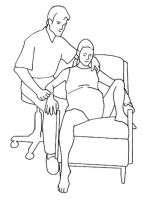

**Fig. 5.10** Asymmetrical sitting.

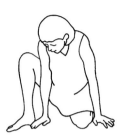

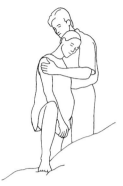

**Fig. 5.11** Asymmetrical kneeling to push.

**Fig. 5.12** Asymmetrical standing.

### *Lateral positions*

For the woman who is exhausted or restricted to bed (Fig. 5.13), sidelying and the exaggerated Sims (semi-prone) positions are good alternatives to the dorsal or semi-sitting positions. If the fetus is thought to be OP, the woman should lie on:

- the *same* side as the posterior occiput if *sidelying* (Fig. 5.14)
- the side *opposite* the posterior or transverse occiput if in *exaggerated Sims (semi-prone)* (Fig. 5.15).

See the explanation of the different effects of the sidelying and semi-prone positions in Chapter 4.

**5**

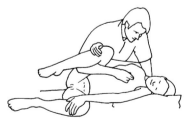

**Fig. 5.13** Lateral pushing.

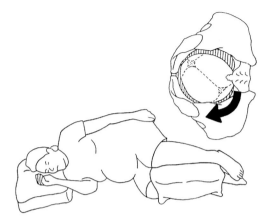

**Fig. 5.14** Woman in pure sidelying on the 'correct' side, with fetal back 'toward the bed'. If fetus is ROP, woman lies on her right side. Gravity pulls fetal occiput and trunk toward ROT.

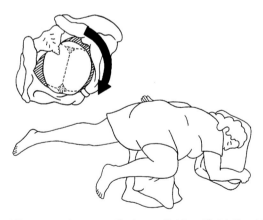

**Fig. 5.15** Woman semi-prone on the 'correct' side, with fetal back 'toward the ceiling'. If fetus is ROP, the semi-prone woman lies on her left side. Gravity pulls fetus occiput and trunk toward ROT, then ROA.

### *Supported squat or 'dangle' positions*

In these the woman is supported under her arms, with no weight-bearing by her legs or feet (Figs 5.16, 5.17). These are the only positions in which the woman is supported from her upper body. We propose the following mechanisms to explain how the dangle positions enhance the fetus's position:

- The woman's own body weight lengthens her trunk by providing traction to her spinal column. This position provides more vertical space for the fetus to maneuver. Most second-stage positions require that the woman flex her trunk and neck, to add pressure to the fundus and promote descent of the fetus. However, this added pressure may not help if the head will not fit because it is asynclitic or deflexed. The dangle positions offer room for the head to reposition itself.

- Furthermore, the dangle positions are almost totally absent of external pressures on the pelvis, such as those that occur when the woman is sitting or lying down, or when her joints are stretched, which occurs when she squats or pulls her legs back. An absence of such external pressures, in cases where the fetal head appears to be 'stuck,' may cause the pressure from the fetal head to change the shape of the pelvic basin as needed for rotation, allowing the fetus to find the path of least resistance through the pelvis.

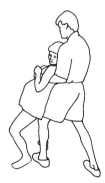

**Fig. 5.16**  Supported squat.

(a)                                        (b)

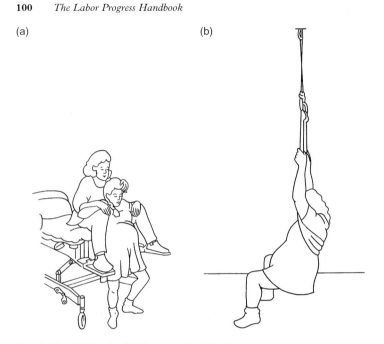

**Fig. 5.17**   (a) Dangle. (b) Dangle with birth sling.

### *Other strategies*

The *pelvic press* is sometimes helpful in cases of deep transverse arrest, occiput posterior, or a 'tight fit' in the second stage, as a method to increase midpelvic and outlet dimensions to make room for fetal rotation and descent[25]. (See Fig. 5.18a, b and also the Toolkit, Chapter 6, page 161, for a description of the pelvic press.)

Please note that the pelvic press is not the same as the 'double hip squeeze.' The main difference between the two is the placement of the hands. The pelvic press is used to enlarge the pelvic outlet in the second stage; the double hip squeeze is used to relieve back pain at any time in labor.

A variety of movements may help rotate the fetus. See Chapter 6 for pelvic rocking (Fig. 5.19 and page 152), lunging (Fig. 5.20 and page 154), slow dancing (Fig. 5.21a and page 157), and swaying on a ball (Fig. 5.21b and page 162).

Because extreme back pain often accompanies fetal malposition, measures to relieve this pain should be used as needed (Figs 5.22–5.31). If the back pain remains tolerable, the woman may have more patience to await fetal rotation and descent. See the Toolkit, Chapter 7, for explanations of these measures.

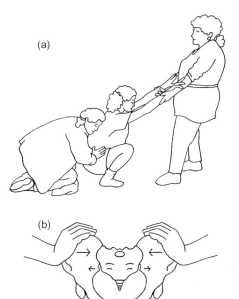

**Fig. 5.18** (a) Pelvic press. (b) Detail of pelvic press.

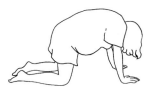

**Fig. 5.19** Pelvic rocking.

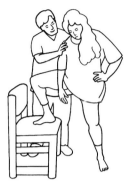

**Fig. 5.20**    Standing lunge.

(a)                                (b)

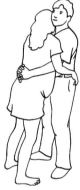

**5**

**Fig. 5.21**    (a) Slow dancing. (b) Swaying on a ball.

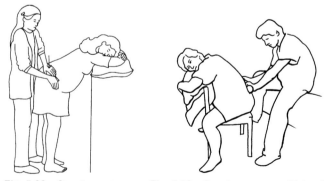

**Fig. 5.22**    Counterpressure.    **Fig. 5.23**    Counterpressure with tennis balls.

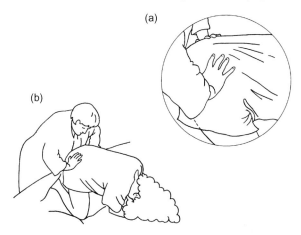

**Fig. 5.24**    (a) Detail of double hip squeeze. (b) Double hip squeeze.

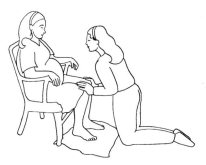

**Fig. 5.25**    Knee press – woman seated.

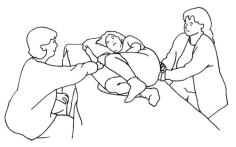

**Fig. 5.26**    Lateral knee press – woman on her side.

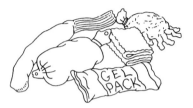

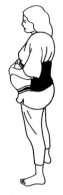

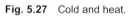

**Fig. 5.27** Cold and heat.

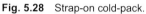

**Fig. 5.28** Strap-on cold-pack.

(a)

(b)

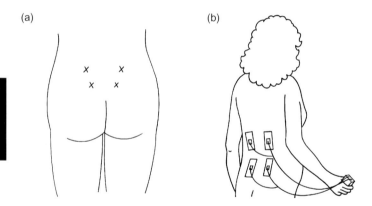

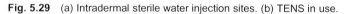

**Fig. 5.29** (a) Intradermal sterile water injection sites. (b) TENS in use.

**5**

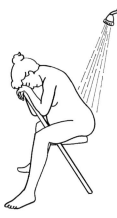

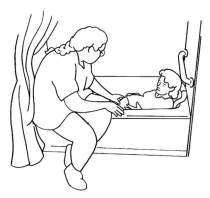

**Fig. 5.30** Shower to relieve back pain.

**Fig. 5.31** Bath to relieve back pain.

## Manual interventions to reposition the OP fetus

Manual rotation of a persistent occiput posterior is a technique described years ago by Hamlin[26] and by Pritchard and MacDonald[27], and recently revived by Davis[25]. Davis describes ways to disengage the fetal head slightly and rotate the head and trunk to anterior (or, if necessary, direct OP) to facilitate descent (Chart 5.5).

Such techniques involve slightly dislodging the fetal head manually per vagina and rotating it to OA, or rotating the woman while holding the fetal head to keep it from rotating. Potential risks of such techniques include cord prolapse or compression, but the incidence of success and of risks has not been documented. It is beyond the scope of this book to describe such techniques as they are not used as 'early interventions.' The reader is referred to the references for further discussion.

**5**

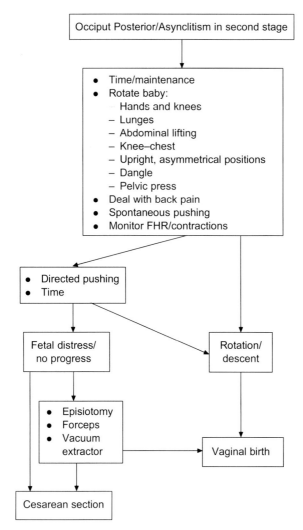

Occiput Posterior/Asynclitism in second stage

- Time/maintenance
- Rotate baby:
    - Hands and knees
    - Lunges
    - Abdominal lifting
    - Knee–chest
    - Upright, asymmetrical positions
    - Dangle
    - Pelvic press
- Deal with back pain
- Spontaneous pushing
- Monitor FHR/contractions

- Directed pushing
- Time

Fetal distress/
no progress

Rotation/
descent

- Episiotomy
- Forceps
- Vacuum
  extractor

Vaginal birth

Cesarean section

**Chart 5.5**

## Early interventions for suspected persistent asynclitism

Normally at the onset of labor the fetal head is in asynclitism (angled so that one parietal bone is presenting), which facilitates entry of the head into the pelvic basin. This usually resolves spontaneously to synclitism as the fetus moves lower in the pelvis. However, persistent asynclitism in the second stage may interfere with flexion, rotation, molding and descent of the fetal head. A caput often forms over one parietal bone.

Extra time and specific interventions encourage the fetus to shift into a more synclitic position. If the caregiver suspects persistent asynclitism, changing the woman's position may assist labor progress in three ways:

(1) Shifting the woman may shift the fetus's weight so its position resolves.
(2) Changing the woman's position may alter the shape of her pelvis slightly, allowing more room for the angle of the fetal head to shift.
(3) Having the woman take a position that elongates her torso (i.e. the dangle and supported squat) may give the fetus room enough to 'wiggle' out of asynclitism. See page 145 for a complete explanation.

5

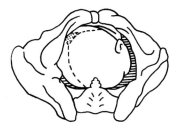
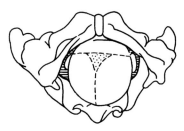

**Fig. 5.32**  Asynclitic fetus in occiput anterior.    **Fig. 5.33**  OA in synclitism.

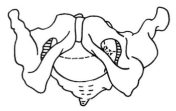

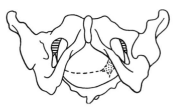

**Fig. 5.34**   Asynclitic fetus in occiput transverse.

**Fig. 5.35**   OT in synclitism.

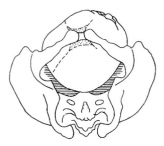

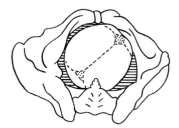

**Fig. 5.36**   Asynclitic fetus in right occiput posterior.

**Fig. 5.37**   Right OP in synclitism.

### Positions and movements for persistent asynclitism in second stage

In general, the same positions and movements and back pain relief techniques in Chapter 4, page 52 for persistent OP/OT are useful when the fetus is in a persistent asynclitic position. (See the Toolkit, Chapter 6 for information on specifics). Specifically, pelvic press and the dangle and supported squat positions may be especially helpful when the fetus is thought to be asynclitic during the second stage. Success with these positions will be influenced by the degree of engagement of the fetal head and the fit between fetal head and woman's pelvis.

### Manual repositioning of the asynclitic fetal head

Doctors and midwives (not maternity nurses or doulas) sometimes try to correct asynclitism manually by dislodging the fetal head and repositioning it so that the sagittal suture line is centered[25]. The technique requires further study of effectiveness and safety.

## If cephalo-pelvic disproportion (CPD) or macrosomia is suspected

When second stage is slow and there is doubt whether the baby will fit through the woman's pelvis, a variety of factors may contribute. These include the size of the fetal head, the size and shape of the woman's pelvis, the position of the fetus, and the woman's ability to move around during labor.

### *The influence of time on CPD*

Many suspected cases of CPD actually involve fetuses who are subtly malpositioned (asynclitic, deflexed, occiput transverse or posterior), who will fit well through the pelvis once the malposition has been resolved. The shape of the woman's pelvis is also a consideration. The woman may need to try pushing in a variety of positions to find the ones that optimize descent. Resolving problems of position or fit often requires extra time.

Many large fetal heads will mold and fit safely through the pelvis, but molding takes time. In the absence of fetal or maternal distress, time can be an ally, not an enemy, in allowing labor progress to take place.

Some midwives and doctors have strict expectations for an acceptable rate of progress in descent. If progress falls behind the expected rate, they initiate interventions such as oxytocin, fundal pressure, episiotomy, forceps, vacuum extraction, or cesarean delivery. Others, however, prefer to exercise patience and less aggressive interventions as long as woman and fetus appear to be doing well.

5

---

**Note: Ultrasound predictions of fetal size**

Ultrasound measurements of fetal weight and head size are not always reliable. For babies weighing over 4000 g (8 lb 13 oz), they can err by 10% (almost a pound) in either direction[28]. Furthermore, even accurate estimates of fetal head size and weight do not predict the capacity of the fetal head or the pelvis to mold to accommodate safe passage of the fetus.

## Positions for 'possible CPD' second stage

As stated above, 'suspected CPD' often results from fetal malpositions, rather than from a true excess of the diameters of the fetal head over the diameters of the pelvic basin. Therefore, it makes sense to encourage the woman to try positions and movements that might resolve an OP, OT, or asynclitic position (Figs 5.38–5.48). See also Fig. 5.17b, page 100.

See Chapter 6 for a discussion of these positions and movements.

Toilet-sitting and hydrotherapy may also enhance progress (Figs 5.49, 5.50).

Encourage movements that adapt pelvic size and shape and encourage fetal descent (Figs 5.51–5.55). See pp. 16–18 for notes on movement and why it helps.

*Note:* To master the technique of the lunge, see the instructions on page 154 before teaching it to the woman in labor.

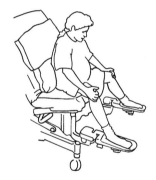

**Fig. 5.38**   Sitting upright to push.

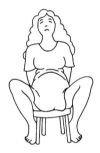

**Fig. 5.39**   Pushing on a low stool.

(a)

(b)

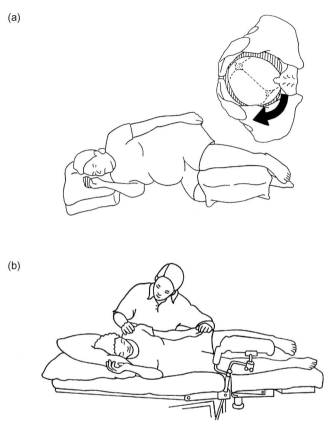

**Fig. 5.40** Woman with OP fetus in pure sidelying on the 'correct' side, with fetal back toward the bed. If fetus is ROP, woman lies on her right side. Gravity pulls fetal head and trunk toward OT.

*Note:* Fetal position is often difficult to ascertain, even with vaginal exams that include palpation of the suture lines of the fetal skull. These exams are often very painful for the woman, and not all that reliable. Other less invasive signs (back pain findings from Leopold's man-euvres, location of heart tones, and shape of the woman's abdomen) often suggest the direction of the fetal occiput.

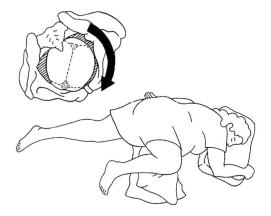

**Fig. 5.41** Woman semi-prone on the 'correct' side, with fetal back 'toward the ceiling'. If fetus is ROP, the semi-prone woman lies on her left side. Gravity pulls fetal head and trunk toward ROT, then ROA.

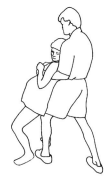

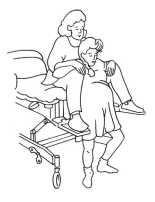

**Fig. 5.42** Supported squat.　　　**Fig. 5.43** Dangle.

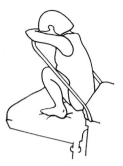

**Fig. 5.44**   Squat with bar.

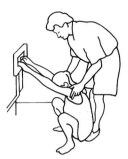

**Fig. 5.45**   Squat with bed rail.

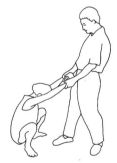

**Fig. 5.46**   Partner squat.

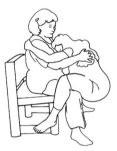

**Fig. 5.47**   Lap squat, two people.

**5**

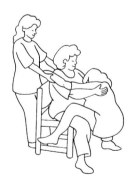

**Fig. 5.48**   Three-person lap squat.

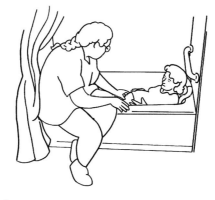

**Fig. 5.49**   Bath.

**5**

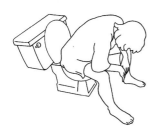

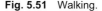

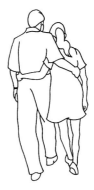

**Fig. 5.50**   Sitting forward on toilet.     **Fig. 5.51**   Walking.

(a) 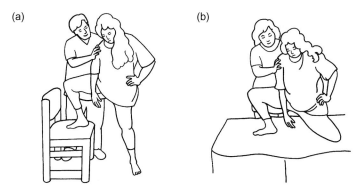 (b)

**Fig. 5.52** (a) Standing lunge. (b) Kneeling lunge.

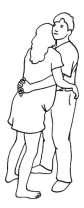

**Fig. 5.53** Slow dancing.　　　　**Fig. 5.54** Stair climbing.

**5**

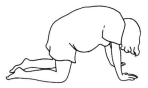

**Fig. 5.55** Pelvic rocking – back rounded into flexion.

### *The use of dorsal positions*

Dorsal positions are the most commonly suggested positions for the second stage today. In fact, many women spend the entire second stage in a dorsal or semi-sitting position (Figs 5.56 and 5.57a, b), even though they would probably use a variety of positions, including upright ones, if given a choice[15]. Though dorsal positions are convenient for caregivers to view the perineum easily, and to perform vaginal exams, episiotomy, vacuum extraction, and forceps, there are some problems associated with these positions:

- The woman's body weight on the bed creates pressure on her sacrum and coccyx, which reduces the anteroposterior diameter of the pelvic outlet[29]. Compare parts (a) and (b) of Fig. 5.58.
- The effects of gravity in promoting descent are lost with supine or any recumbent positions.
- Maternal supine hypotension is caused by the weight of the uterus on the inferior vena cava and aorta, which leads to a reduction in venous return and cardiac output. The fetus may then experience hypoxia due to the concomitant decrease in blood flow to the placenta and resulting reduction in oxygen supply to the fetus.
- Besides supine hypotension, the weight of the uterus along the spinal column reduces the angle of the uterus with the spine, resulting in poor alignment of the fetus with the pelvis[30] (Fig. 2.2).

**5**

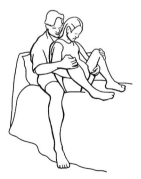

**Fig. 5.56**   Semi-sitting to push.

(a)

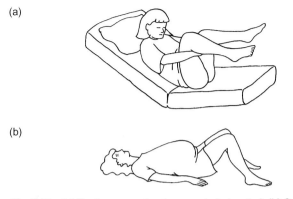

(b)

**Fig. 5.57** (a) Supine, upper trunk somewhat elevated. (b) Supine, knees flexed.

(a)                                    (b)

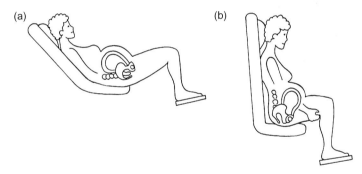

**Fig. 5.58** (a) Woman reclining. Adapted from reference 29. (b) Woman upright. Adapted from reference 29.

With persistent OP, persistent asynclitism, or other malpositions, the woman should be encouraged to do most of her pushing in positions other than supine or semi-sitting.

It is ironic that two widely prescribed practices for second stage – prolonged breath-holding and straining, and the supine position – are at least partly responsible for the frequently observed fetal bradycardias and prolonged second stage that have led caregivers to believe that the duration of the second stage must be curtailed. The further irony is that if laboring women were encouraged to behave instinctually, they would not lie on their backs, nor would they use prolonged breath-holding and straining; thus, much of the worrisome 'fetal distress' in the second stage would not occur.

### Use of the exaggerated lithotomy position

Notwithstanding what was stated above in relation to disadvantages of dorsal positions, there are occasions when one particular dorsal position – the exaggerated lithotomy (McRoberts') position – may succeed in promoting descent when no other position does. When the woman has been unable to bring her baby beneath the pubic symphysis in any other position, this problem may in some cases be resolved by use of an exaggerated lithotomy position (in which the woman lies flat on her back with her knees drawn back so that her buttocks are lifted slightly off the bed, and her hips are in a very flexed, abducted position) (Figs 5.59 and 5.60). This position passively rotates the pubic arch upward toward the mother's head and brings the pelvic inlet perpendicular to the maximum expulsive force[31,32].

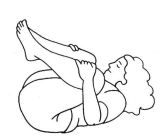

**Fig. 5.59**   Exaggerated lithotomy position.

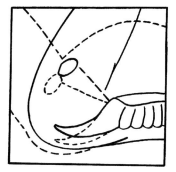

**Fig. 5.60**   Exaggerated lithotomy (detail).

Such a position may facilitate the passage of the fetal head beneath the pubic arch. In particularly persistent delays in descent this benefit may outweigh the disadvantages of supine hypotension and loss of any gravity advantage. Such a position is combined with maximal breath-holding and straining. It is worth trying when operative delivery is anticipated.

## If emotional dystocia is suspected

Emotional distress sometimes underlies a lack of progress in the second stage. Much of the information in Chapters 2 and 4 on the physiology of emotional dystocia and on measures to alleviate it during the first stage of labor will also apply to the second stage. In addition, these other factors might trigger emotional distress in the second stage:

- fatigue or exhaustion, which can lead to hopelessness or anxiety
- the intense sensations of second stage or of manual stretching of the vagina. These sensations may be especially frightening if the woman has been sexually abused in the past, as they may trigger flashbacks to the abuse
- fear of behaving inappropriately or offensively (making noise, passing stool while pushing)
- the immediacy of the birth and the responsibility of parenting the child, especially if her own parents were dysfunctional, or she has relinquished a child for adoption, or had a child removed from her care
- fear for the baby's well-being, especially if a sibling or a previous child died around birth or had another adverse outcome
- the loss of privacy, lack of modesty when surrounded by strangers watching her perineum
- previous cesarean during second stage
- thoughtless or unkind treatment by loved ones or caregiver during labor.

**5**

One common response to such fears in the second stage is to 'hold back' while pushing. The woman may be pushing hard, but not effectively. Sometimes she actually contracts her pelvic floor muscles and buttocks as she pushes with her diaphragm and abdominal muscles. Tension in the perineum and constriction of the anus while pushing indicate that the woman is holding back.

It is important not to confuse 'holding back' with the normal confusion many women have when they first begin to push. It is normal for the woman to have to experiment a bit in order to discover how to push effectively. This is particularly true for women who do not initially have a strong urge to push. In such cases, it may be best for them to rest and await a stronger urge to push.

Whatever fears or anxieties cause the woman to hold back, she probably cannot simply 'snap out of it.' However, those around her may be able to address and alleviate her fears. The measures described in Chapter 3 may help, along with the following:

- Encourage the woman to express her feelings. Ask her, 'What was going through your mind during that last contraction?' Listen to her, acknowledge and validate her concerns, and try to give appropriate reassurance, encouragement, or information and suggestions. Often, all the woman needs is a chance to express her concerns. She needs to know that she is being heard, that her fears are normal, and that she will get through this event. Even normal events can be very troublesome to a woman.

- Sometimes, when it is clear to all including the woman that there is a delay, asking her, 'Why do you think labor has slowed down?' reveals useful information. Answers such as, 'I can't push right,' or, 'The baby doesn't want to come out,' might indicate emotional dystocia.

- Provide appropriate information. For example, if the woman is afraid of having a bowel movement as she pushes (and it is too late for her to go to the bathroom), she can be reassured that passing stool indicates that she is pushing effectively, that this is a common event, that any fecal material will be quickly wiped away and disposed of.

- If she is afraid she will 'rip' or split apart while pushing, reassure her that, by relaxing her perineum or letting the baby come, it actually stretches better and a tear is less likely. Also, if fetal condition permits, let her try a few contractions without pushing. 'Let's try breathing through this next one,' so that she feels she has some options during this frightening time.

- Give the woman time to adjust to the intense sensations and emotions of second stage. Avoid creating a sense of rushing. There is usually no need for the caregiver to raise his or her voice.

- Encourage the woman to relax her perineum between contractions and let it bulge during contractions. The application of hot compresses (washcloths soaked in hot water, wrung out) to the perineum often feels good and promotes relaxation.

- Encourage the woman to push as if she is blowing up a balloon. Pushing in this manner sometimes causes the pelvic floor to bulge.

- Have the woman try pushing while sitting on the toilet. If she is worried about passing stool, the toilet is a reassuring place to be. Toilet-sitting also elicits the conditioned response of releasing the pelvic floor. Whoever is responsible for the woman's care can monitor what the woman is feeling. If the woman feels that the baby is coming, she will need to get off the toilet for a more appropriate delivery site.

If the woman is pushing in a 'diffuse' manner, see pages 86–8.

## REFERENCES

1. Simkin, P. (1984) Active and physiologic management of second stage: a review and hypothesis. In: *Episiotomy and the Second Stage of Labor*. Kitzinger, S. and Simkin, P. (eds). Pennypress, Seattle.
2. Simkin, P. (1989) *The Birth Partner*. Harvard Common Press, Boston.
3. Kitzinger, S. (1996) *The Complete Book of Pregnancy and Childbirth*. Alfred A. Knopf, New York.
4. Friedman, E.A. (1978) Normal labor. In: *Labor: Clinical Evaluation and Management*, 2nd edition. Appleton Century Crofts, New York.
5. Cohen, W.R. and Friedman, E.A. (1983) Dysfunctional labor. In: *Management of Labor*. University Park Press, Baltimore.
6. Vasicka, A., Kumaresan, P., Han, G.S. and Kumaresan, M. (1978) Plasma oxytocin in initiation of labor. *Am. J. Obstet. Gynecol.* **130(3)**, 263–73.
7. Fuchs, A.R., Romero, R., Keefe, D., Parra, M., Oyarzun, E. and Behnke, E. (1991) Oxytocin secretion and human parturition: Pulse frequency and duration increase during spontaneous labor in women. *Am. J. Obstet. Gynecol.* **165(5, Part 1)**, 1515–23.
8. Beynon, C.L. (1957) The normal second stage of labour: A plea for reform in its conduct. *J. Obstet. Gynaecol. Brit. Commonw.* **64(6)**, 815–20.
9. Sleep, J., Roberts, J. and Chalmers, I. (1989) Care during the second stage of labour. In: *Effective Care in Pregnancy and Childbirth*, vol. 2. Chalmers, I., Enkin, M. and Keirse, M.J.N.C. (eds). Oxford University Press, Oxford.
10. BMA/RPSGB (1997) *British National Formulary*, British Medical Association and The Royal Pharmaceutical Society of Great Britain Number 33, Pharmaceutical Press, London.
11. Rosevear, S. and Stirrat, G. (1996) *The Handbook of Obstetric Management*. Blackwell Scientific, Oxford.
12. Roberts, J. and Woolley, D. (1996) A second look at the second stage of labor. *JOGNN* **25(5)**, 415–23.
13. Bing, E. (1994) Personal communication.
14. Aldrich, C.J., D'Antona, D., Spencer, J.A.D., Wyatt, J.S., Peebles, D.M., Delpy, D.T., Reynolds, E.O.R. (1995) The effect of maternal pushing on

**5**

fetal cerebral oxygenation and blood volume during the second stage of labour. *Br. J. Obstet. Gynaecol.* **102**, 448–53.

15. Carlson, J.M., Diehl, J.A., Sachtleben-Murray, M., McRae, M., Fenwick, L. and Friedman, E.A. (1986) Maternal position during parturition in normal labor. *Obstet. Gynecol.* **68(4)**, 443–7.

16. Fuller, B.F., Roberts, J.E. and McKay, S. (1993) Acoustical analysis of maternal sounds during the second stage of labor. *Applied Nurs Res.* **6**, 7–13.

17. Caldeyro-Barcia, R. (1986) Influence of maternal bearing-down efforts during second stage on fetal well-being. In: *Episiotomy and the Second Stage of Labor.* Kitzinger, S. and Simkin, P. (eds). Pennypress, Seattle.

18. Enkin, M., Keirse, M.J.N.C., Renfrew, M. and Neilson, J. (1995) Control of pain in labour. In: *A Guide to Effective Care in Labour*, 2nd edition. Oxford University Press, Oxford.

19. Bonica, J.J., Miller, F.C. and Parmley, T.H. (1995) Anatomy and physiology of the forces of parturition. In: *Principles and Practice of Obstetric Analgesia and Anesthesia*, 2nd edition. Bonica, J.J. and McDonald, J.S. (eds). Williams & Wilkins, Philadelphia.

20. Spiby, H. (1993) Early vs. late pushing with epidural anesthesia in 2nd stage of labour, Cochrane Updates on Disk, Oxford: Update Software, Disk Issue 1.

21. Maresh, M., Choong, K. and Beard, R.W. (1983) Delayed pushing with lumbar epidural analgesia in labour. *Br. J. Obstet. Gynaecol.* **90**, 623–7.

22. Committee on Obstetrics: Maternal and fetal medicine (1988). Obstetric forceps. *ACOG Committee Opinion No. 59.*

23. Vause, S., Congdon, H.M. and Thornton, J.G. (1998) Immediate and delayed pushing in the second stage of labour for nulliparous women with epidural analgesia: A randomized controlled trial. *Br. J. Obstet. Gynaecol.* **105** (2), 186–8.

24. Friedman, E.A. (1995) Dystocia and "failure to progress" in labor. In: *Cesarean Section: Guidelines for Appropriate Utilization.* Flamm, B.L. and Quilligan, E.J. (eds). Springer-Verlag, New York (quote from p. 36).

25. Davis, E. (1997) *Heart and Hands: A Caregiver's Guide to Pregnancy and Birth*, 3rd edition. Celestial Arts, Berkeley.

26. Hamlin, R.H.J. (1959) *Stepping Stones to Labour Ward Diagnosis.* Rigby Ltd, Adelaide.

27. Pritchard, J.A. and MacDonald, P.C. (1980) *Williams Obstetrics*, 16th edition. Appleton Century Crofts, New York.

28. Winn, H.N. and Hobbins, J.C. (1995) Fetal macrosomia. In: *Cesarean Section: Guidelines for Appropriate Utilization.* Flamm, B.L. and Quilligan, E.J. (eds). Springer-Verlag, New York.

29. Fenwick, L. and Simkin, P. (1987) Maternal position to prevent or alleviate dystocia in labor. *Clin. Obstet. Gynecol.* **30**, 83–9.

30. Sutton, J. and Scott, P. (1994) Optimal fetal positioning: a midwifery

**5**

approach to increasing the number of normal births. *MIDIRS Midwifery Digest* **4** (3), 283–6.

31. Smeltzer, J.S. (1986) Prevention and management of shoulder dystocia. *Clin. Obstet. Gynecol.* **29** (2), 299–308.

32. Sweet, B.R. and Tiran, D. (eds) (1997) *Mayes' Widwifery*. Baillière Tindall, London.

5

# Chapter 6

# The Labor Progress Toolkit: Part 1. Maternal Positions and Movements

6

This Toolkit, which consists of Chapters 6 (Maternal Positions and Movements) and 7 (Comfort Measures), contains descriptions of numerous techniques for enhancing labor progress and maintaining comfort in both the first and second stages.

Many of these techniques are designed to improve the biomechanical forces of labor: the powers, passage, and passenger. They include such techniques as the woman's use of her own body; the use of props to support the woman in particular positions or movements; and the use of pressure or physical support by another person.

Many techniques are designed to reduce pain and enhance relaxation without using pain medications. When pain is reduced, the woman's tolerance of a prolonged labor is improved, which allows more time for the use of primary interventions. Without drugs, there are fewer, if any, side effects that might interfere with labor progress or adversely affect woman or baby.

Many reduce anxiety, fear, and distress, all of which may contribute to excessive catecholamine production, which sometimes results in slowing of uterine contractions as well as fetal stress.

## MATERNAL POSITIONS

This section contains descriptions of positions and specific features of each. We have arranged the positions in categories. The positions in each category cause similar physical changes. For example:

- Semi-sitting and sidelying positions are restful and gravity neutral. They may help an exhausted woman save her energy, especially if she has been up and walking for a long period. Also, if progress is rapid, neutralizing gravity may slow the labor to a more manageable pace.
- Upright positions take advantage of gravity to apply the presenting part to the cervix, improve the quality of the contractions, and enhance the descent of the fetus[1,2].
- Positions in which the woman leans forward tend to enhance fetal rotation and reduce back pain[3,4].
- Asymmetrical positions in which the woman elevates one leg tend to enhance rotation and reduce back pain.
- The exaggerated lithotomy position, used for several contractions in the second stage, may facilitate the passage of a 'stuck baby' beneath the pubic symphysis.

**6**

- Dorsal positions tend to cause supine hypotension and increase back pain. Contractions are more frequent and painful, yet less likely to improve labor progress[1].

## Sidelying positions

***When:*** During first and second stages.

***How:*** *For pure sidelying:* Woman lies on side with both hips and knees flexed and a pillow between her legs, or with her upper leg raised and supported (Figs 6.1–6.3).

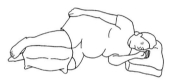

**Fig. 6.1** Sidelying.

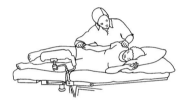

**Fig. 6.2** Sidelying, leg in leg rest.

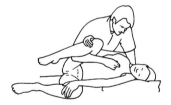

**Fig. 6.3** Sidelying to push.

**6**

*For exaggerated Sims or semi-prone:* Woman lies on side with lower arm behind (or in front of) her trunk, her lower leg extended, and her upper leg flexed more than 90° and supported by one or two pillows. She rolls partly toward her front (Figs 6.4, 6.5).

See below for information on which side the woman should lie on.

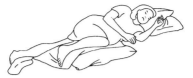

**Fig. 6.4** Semi-prone, lower arm forward.

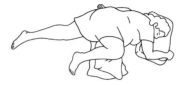

**Fig. 6.5** Semi-prone, lower arm behind her.

### *What these positions do*

- Allow tired women to rest
- Are safe if pain medications have been used
- Are gravity neutral (can be used with a very rapid first or second stage)
- May relieve hemorrhoids
- May resolve fetal heart rate problems, if due to cord compression or supine hypotension
- Help lower high blood pressure (especially the left lateral positions)
- May promote progress when alternated with walking
- Avoid pressure on sacrum (unlike sitting and supine positions)
- In second stage, because there is no pressure on the sacrum (as there is with sitting) these positions allow posterior movement of the sacrum as the fetus descends.
- May enhance rotation of an occiput posterior (OP) baby.

*Note:* Gravity effects are different when a woman is in pure sidelying or semi-prone.

If sidelying, the woman with an OP fetus should lie on the *same* side as the fetal occiput and back ('baby's back toward bed'; Fig. 6.6). This helps shift the fetus from OP to OT. Ask the woman with an OP fetus to lie on the same side as the occiput for 15–30 minutes to encourage rotation from OP to OT; then ask her to change to kneeling and leaning forward for 15 to 30 minutes (to encourage rotation from OT to occiput anterior). As can be seen in Fig. 6.7, lying on the side opposite the fetal occiput actually utilizes gravity to take the fetus into direct OP.

If the woman is semi-prone ('exaggerated Sims'), she should lie on the side *opposite* the fetal occiput ('baby's back toward ceiling', Fig. 6.8) for at least 15 to 30 minutes. In this position, her pelvis is rotated so that the front of it is pointing more toward the bed than with straight sidelying. This alters the effects of gravity so that the fetal trunk is encouraged to rotate to transverse and then to anterior.

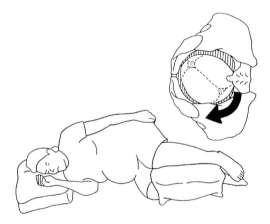

**Fig. 6.6** Woman in pure sidelying on the 'correct' side, with fetal back 'toward the bed'. If fetus is ROP, woman lies on her right side. Gravity pulls fetal occiput and trunk toward ROT.

6

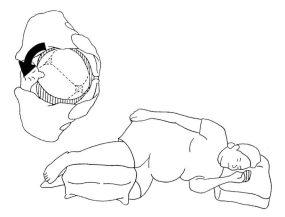

**Fig. 6.7** Woman in pure sidelying on the 'wrong' side for an ROP fetus. Fetal back is toward the ceiling. Gravity pulls fetal occiput and trunk toward OP.

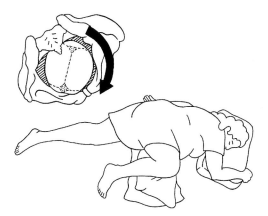

**Fig. 6.8** Woman semi-prone on the 'correct' side, with fetal back 'toward the ceiling'. If fetus is ROP, the semi-prone woman lies on her side. Gravity pulls fetal occiput and trunk toward ROT, then ROA.

**6**

### When to use sidelying positions

- As long as labor continues to progress well and the woman wants it
- When supine hypotension occurs
- When the woman has been given narcotics or an epidural
- When the woman has pregnancy-induced hypertension
- When the woman finds it comfortable in first or second stage
- When the woman is tired
- In second stage, if hemorrhoids are painful in dorsal positions.

### When not to use sidelying positions

- When the woman objects, due to increased pain or preference for another position. However, if it is explained that this position may improve labor progress, the woman may be willing to try it.
- When a gravity advantage is needed to aid descent, especially if second stage progress has slowed
- When she has been in sidelying for more than an hour without progress.

## Semi-sitting

**When:** During first and second stages.
**How:** Woman sits with trunk at >45° angle with bed (Figs 6.9a, 6.10).

### What this position does

- Provides some gravity advantage, when compared with supine
- May be better than supine for:
  - increasing pelvic inlet dimensions
  - improving oxygenation of fetus
- Is an easy position to assume
- Pressure on sacrum and coccyx may impair pelvic joint movement.

**6**

### When to use semi-sitting positions

- If progress is good, and woman prefers it
- When the woman needs rest
- When an epidural is in place
- For caregiver's convenience during second stage in viewing perineum

(a)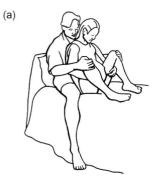

(b)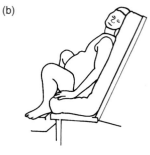

(c)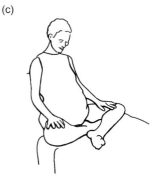

(d)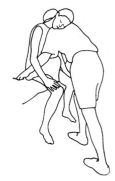

(e)

(f)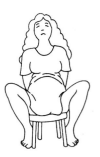

**Fig. 6.9** (a) Semi-sitting to push. (b) Sitting upright on bed. (c) Tailor sitting. (d) Sitting upright with partner support. (e) Sitting upright to push. (f) Pushing on a low stool.

### *When not to use semi-sitting positions*

- With occiput posterior fetus
- If fetus is in distress
- If woman has hypertension and this position exacerbates it
- When the woman objects, due to increased pain or preference for another position. However, once it is explained that this position might improve labor progress, the woman may be willing to try it.

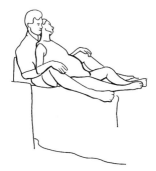

**Fig. 6.10**    Semi-sitting.

## Sitting upright

*When:* During first and second stages.
*How:* Woman sits straight up on bed, chair or stool (Figs 6.9b–6.9f).

### *What this position does*

- Provides gravity advantage
- Allows a tired woman to rest, if she is well supported
- Allows for placement of hot or cold packs on shoulders, low back, lower abdomen
- Enables woman to rock or sway if rocking chair or birth ball is used.

### *When to use upright sitting, positions*

- When woman needs to rest
- When woman has backache

- When woman finds it comfortable in first or second stage
- When active labor progress has slowed; sitting up is especially beneficial if her knees are lower than her hips[5].

### When not to use upright sitting positions

- When the woman objects, due to increased pain or a preference for another position. However, if it is explained that there is a chance that this position will improve labor progress, the woman may be willing to try it
- When fetal heart rate is compromised in that position.

## Sitting leaning forward with support

**When:** During first and second stages.
**How:** Woman sits with feet firmly placed and leans forward, arms resting on thighs or on a prop in front of her (Figs 6.11 and 6.13b); or she straddles a chair or toilet and rests her upper body on the back (Figs 6.12–6.13a).

### What this position does

- Provides gravity advantage
- Is restful if woman is well supported
- Relieves backache
- May enhance rotation from occiput posterior (when compared with supine, semi-sitting)
- Aligns fetus with pelvis (Fig. 2.2)[6]
- Enlarges pelvic inlet (when compared with supine)
- Allows easy access for backrub.

**6**

### When to use sitting and leaning forward

- If woman is semi-reclining and labor is not progressing, to shift the weight of the fetal torso off the woman's spine
- When the woman has backache
- When woman finds it comfortable in first or second stage
- When active labor progress has slowed.

### *When not to use sitting and leaning forward*

- When the woman objects, due to increased pain or a preference for another position. However, if it is explained that this position may improve labor progress, the woman may be willing to try it
- If labor progress does not improve in this position.

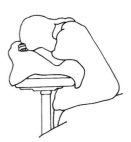

**Fig. 6.11** Sitting, leaning on tray table.

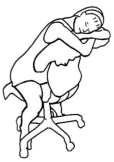

**Fig. 6.12** Straddling a chair.

(a)

(b)

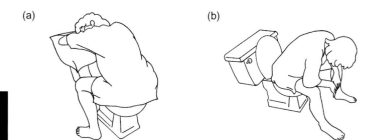

**Fig. 6.13** (a) Straddling a toilet. (b) Sitting forward on toilet.

## Standing, leaning forward

*When:* During first and second stage.
*How:* Woman stands and leans on partner, on a raised bed, over a birth ball placed on the bed, or on a counter (Figs 6.14–6.17).

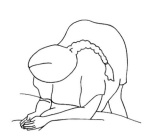

**Fig. 6.14** Standing, leaning forward on bed.

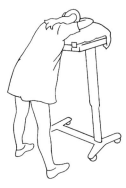

**Fig. 6.15** Standing, leaning on a tray table.

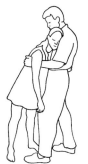

**Fig. 6.16** Standing, leaning on partner.

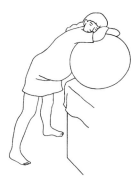

**Fig. 6.17** Standing, leaning on birth ball.

**6**

### *What this position does*

- Provides gravity advantage
- Enlarges pelvic inlet (when compared with supine or sitting)
- Aligns fetus with pelvic inlet[5,6] (Fig. 2.2)
- May promote flexion of fetal head
- May enhance rotation from OP, especially if combined with swaying movements[5]

- Causes contractions to be less painful but more productive than in supine or sitting[1]
- Relieves backache by reducing pressure of the fetal presenting part on the woman's sacrum
- May be easier to maintain than hands and knees position
- If the woman is embraced and supported in the upright position by her partner, the embrace increases her sense of well-being and may reduce catecholamine production
- May increase her urge to push in second stage.

### *When to use standing and leaning forward*

- When labor progress is slow or arrested
- When contractions space out or lose intensity
- When woman has backache
- When woman finds it comfortable in first or second stage.

### *When not to use standing and leaning forward*

- When the woman objects, due to increased pain or a preference for another position. However, if it is explained that this position may improve labor progress, the woman may be willing to try it.
- When birth is imminent, and the attendant does not want to deliver in this position.

## Kneeling, leaning forward with support

*When:* During first and second stages.
*How:* Woman kneels on bed or floor, leaning forward onto back of bed, chair seat, birth ball, or other support (Figs 6.18–6.21).

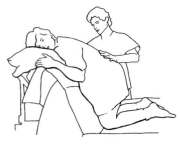

**Fig. 6.18**  Kneeling over back of bed

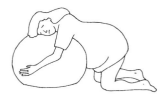

**Fig. 6.19**  Kneeling with a ball.

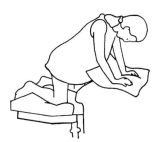 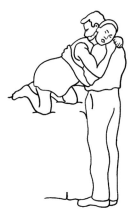

**Fig. 6.20**   Kneeling on foot of bed.   **Fig. 6.21**   Kneeling with partner support to push.

### What this position does

- Provides some gravity advantage
- Aligns fetus with pelvic inlet
- Enlarges pelvic inlet more than sidelying, supine, or sitting
- Allows easy access for back pressure
- Relieves strain on hands and wrists when compared with hands and knees
- Allows easy movement (swaying, rocking)
- May relieve cord compression
- May cause soreness in knees (to prevent this, woman can wear kneepads made for sports or gardening).

### When to use kneeling and leaning forward

- When fetus is occiput posterior
- When woman has backache
- When woman is in a bath or pool
- When fetal distress is noted with supine or sidelying position
- When fetus is at a high station
- If woman finds it comfortable
- To alternate with other positions for backache.

6

### *When not to use kneeling and leaning forward*

- When woman has pain in knees or legs
- If woman is very tired
- When first or second stage is not progressing in the position.

## Hands and knees

***When:*** During first and second stages.

***How:*** Woman kneels (preferably on a padded surface), leans forward and supports herself on either the palms of her hands or her fists (the latter being more tolerable if she has carpal tunnel syndrome). See Fig. 6.22. Knee pads may make her more comfortable.

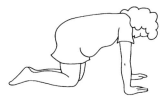

**Fig. 6.22**   Hands and knees.

### *What this position does*

- Aids fetal rotation from OP
- May aid in reducing an anterior lip in late first stage
- Reduces back pain
- Allows swaying, crawling, or rocking motion to promote rotation and increase comfort
- Relieves hemorrhoids
- May resolve fetal heart rate problems, especially if due to cord compression
- Allows easy access for counterpressure or double hip squeeze (pages 182–5)
- Allows access for vaginal exams
- Arms may tire; to relieve, she rests upper body and head on a pile of pillows, chair seat, or birth ball.

### When to use hands and knees

- When woman has backache
- When fetus is occiput posterior
- When woman finds it comfortable in first or second stage
- When an anterior lip slows progress.

### When not to use hands and knees

- When the woman objects, due to increased pain or a preference for another position. However, if it is explained that this position may improve labor progress, the woman may be willing to try it.

## Open knee–chest position

***When:*** During first and second stages.

***How:*** Woman kneels, leans forward to support weight on her hands, then lowers her chest to the floor, so that her buttocks are higher than her chest. In the *open* knee–chest position (Fig. 6.23) her hips are less flexed (>90° angle) than in the usual *closed* knee–chest position (Fig. 6.24). The more open position puts the pelvis at a very different angle from that when the knees are drawn up under her trunk.

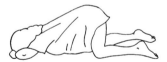

**Fig. 6.23**   Open knee–chest position.

### What this position does

- Protects against fetal distress with prolapsed cord
- If used for 30 to 45 minutes during the latent phase or any time before engagement it allows repositioning of the fetal head. Gravity encourages the fetal head to 'back out' of the pelvis and rotate or flex before re-entering
- May resolve some fetal heart rate problems
- Reduces back pain
- Relieves hemorrhoids
- It is tiring. Pillows and support from the partner makes the position easier.

**6**

### When to use the open knee–chest position

- If there is a prolapsed cord
- When one suspects OP in pre-labor or early labor, as indicated by contractions that are short, frequent, irregular, and painful, especially in the low back, and not accompanied by dilation[7]. This position may be alternated with semi-prone (exaggerated Sims) position. See page 41 for further description.
- When woman has a backache
- When it is necessary for woman to avoid a premature urge to push
- When woman has a swollen cervix or anterior lip
- If caregiver will perform a manual rotation of the posterior head during second stage.

### When not to use the open knee–chest position

- During a normally progressing second stage (works against gravity).

## Closed knee–chest position

***When:*** During first and second stage**s.**
***How:*** Woman kneels, and leans forward, supporting herself on her hands, then lowers her chest to the bed, with her knees and hips flexed and abducted under her abdomen (Fig. 6.24).

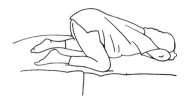

**Fig. 6.24**   Closed knee–chest position.

### What this position does

- Reduces back pain
- Is less strenuous than hands and knees or 'open' knee–chest position (see pages 138–40)

- Spreads ischia, enlarging bispinous and intertuberous diameters
- Relieves hemorrhoids
- May resolve some fetal heart rate problems
- Is an anti-gravity position which may help reduce an anterior lip.

### When to use the closed knee–chest position

- When woman has a backache
- When woman has a swollen cervix or anterior lip
- If there is a prolapsed cord.

### When not to use the closed knee–chest position

- In pre-labor or early labor when rotation is desired (Instead try open knee–chest with hips at >90° angle. See page 139.)
- When the woman objects, due to increased pain or a preference for another position. However, if it is explained that this position may improve labor progress, the woman may be willing to try it
- If woman becomes short of breath, has gastric upset, or other discomfort
- During a normally progressing second stage (works against gravity).

## Asymmetrical upright (standing, kneeling, sitting) positions

**When:** During first and second stages.

**How:** Woman sits, stands, or kneels, with one knee and hip flexed, and foot elevated above the other (Figs 6.25–6.27). Comfort guides woman in which leg to raise. She should try both sides; one side may be much more comfortable than the other; the more comfortable side is probably the one to use.

**6**

### What these positions do

- Exert a mild stretch on adductor muscles of the raised thigh, causing some lateral movement of the ischium, thus increasing pelvic outlet diameter
- May aid rotation from occiput posterior
- Reduce back pain
- Provide gravity advantage

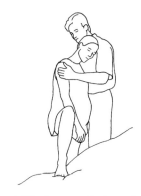

**Fig. 6.25**   Asymmetrical standing.

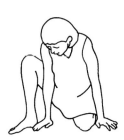

**Fig. 6.26**   Asymmetrical kneeling.

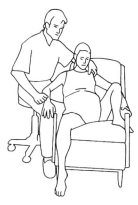

**Fig. 6.27**   Asymmetrical sitting.

6

- Allow woman to 'lunge' in this position, thereby causing the pelvic outlet to widen even more on that side. (See page 154.)

### When to use asymmetrical upright positions

- When woman has backache
- When active labor progress has slowed
- When rotation is desired in first or second stage
- When fetus is suspected to be asynclitic.

### *When not to use asymmetrical upright positions*

- When woman finds that these positions increase pain in her knees, hips, or pubic joint
- When she has an epidural or narcotics that may weaken her legs or impair her balance.

## Squatting

***When:*** Primarily during second stage, but any time the mother finds it comfortable.

***How:*** Woman lowers herself from standing into a squatting position with her feet flat on the floor or bed, using her partner, a squatting bar, other support for balance, if necessary (Figs 6.28–6.30).

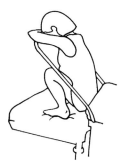

**Fig. 6.28**  Squatting with bar.

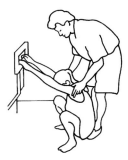

**Fig. 6.29**  Squatting holding bed rail.

**6**

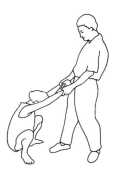

**Fig. 6.30**  Partner squat.

## What this position does

- Provides gravity advantage
- Enlarges pelvic outlet by increasing the intertuberous diameter
- May require less bearing-down effort than horizontal positions
- May enhance urge to push
- May enhance fetal descent
- May relieve backache
- Allows freedom to shift weight for comfort
- Provides mechanical advantage: upper trunk presses on fundus more than in many other positions
- May impede correction of the angle of the head, if the fetus is at a relatively high station and asynclitic. The pressure of the woman's upper torso on the fundus may reduce the space available for the fetus to 'wriggle' into synclitism. (Positions that lengthen the trunk and relax the pelvic joints may be preferable. See supported squat and dangle.) However, if the fetal head is engaged and well-aligned in occiput anterior (OA), squatting may hasten descent.
- If continued for a prolonged period, compresses the blood vessels and nerves located behind the knee joint, impairing circulation and possibly causing entrapment neuropathy. As long as the woman sits back or rises to standing after every contraction or two, such problems are avoided. *Please note:* Women for whom squatting is a customary resting position do not have these potential nerve and circulation problems.

### When to use squatting

- When more space within the pelvis is desired during second stage, especially when fetus is OA
- When descent is inadequate.

### When not to use squatting

- When there is lower extremity joint injury, arthritis, or weakness in legs
- When fetal head has not reached the level of the ischial spines
- When an epidural has caused motor or sensory block in legs.

## Supported squatting positions

***When:*** During second stage.

***How:*** *The supported squat:* During contractions, woman leans with back against partner, who places his or her forearms under her arms and holds her hands, taking all her weight (Fig. 6.31). She stands between contractions.

*The 'Dangle:'* Partner sits on a high bed or counter, feet supported on chairs or footrests, with thighs spread. Woman stands between partner's legs with her back to her partner, and places her flexed arms over partner's thighs. During the contraction she lowers herself, and her partner grips the sides of her chest with his thighs; her full weight is supported by her arms on his thighs and the grip of his thighs on her upper trunk (Fig. 6.32a). She stands between contractions. A 'birth sling', suspended from the ceiling, may also be used to support the woman (Figs 6.32b). The dangle or use of a birth sling is much easier for the partner than the supported squat.

### *What this position does*

- Provides gravity advantage
- Elongates woman's trunk: may help resolve asynclitism by giving fetus more room to renegotiate angle of head in pelvis
- Allows more mobility in pelvic joints than in other positions
- Allows fetal head to 'mold' the woman's pelvis as needed

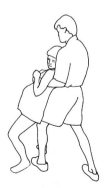

**Fig. 6.31** Supported squat.

6

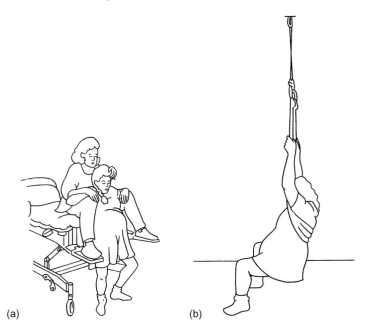

**Fig. 6.32**   (a) Dangle. (b) Dangle with birth sling.

- Enables woman to feel safe and supported by partner, which may reduce catecholamines
- The supported squat requires great strength in the support person, and it is tiring. To make it easier for the partner, he or she may lean back on a wall for support, make sure to maintain a straight back (not lean forward at all), and alternate this with other positions. See also page 99.
- If prolonged, may cause paresthesia (numbness, tingling) in woman's hands, from pressure of partner's arms or thighs in her armpits (causing nerve compression in the brachial plexus). To prevent this, suggest that the woman stand up and lean on her partner between contractions.
- The dangle allows the partner's legs or the birth sling to support all of woman's weight, making it less tiring for the partner than supported squat. (If the partner places his feet directly beneath his

knees, the woman's weight is borne without the partner having to rely totally on muscle strength.)

- The dangle leaves the partner's hands free to stroke or hold woman.

### When to use supported squatting positions

- When more mobility of pelvic joints is needed
- When lengthening of the woman's trunk seems desirable
- In second stage, when fetal head is thought to be large, asynclitic, occiput posterior, or occiput transverse
- When descent is not taking place.

### When not to use supported squatting positions

- When the woman objects, due to increased pain or a preference for another position. However, if it is explained that this position may improve labor progress, the woman may be willing to try it
- When birth is imminent, unless the caregiver has agreed to deliver in this position
- When the woman has an epidural or narcotics that interfere with her balance or the use of her legs
- When no one is available who is strong enough to support the woman or there is no birth sling available.

## Lap squatting

*When:* During second stage.
*How:* Partner sits on armless straight chair; woman sits on partner's lap facing and embracing partner and straddling partner's thighs. Partner embraces her and spreads thighs during contractions, allowing woman's buttocks to sag between, while she keeps from sagging too far by bending her knees over partner's thighs. Partner does not lean forward (Fig. 6.33). Between contractions, partner brings legs together so the woman is sitting up on them. Another person can assist in supporting the woman while she sits on her partner's lap (Fig. 6.34).

### What this position does

- Provides gravity advantage
- Allows woman to rest between contractions, if she is held

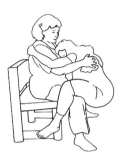
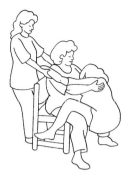

**Fig. 6.33** Two-person lap squat.    **Fig. 6.34** Three-person lap squat.

- Passively enlarges pelvic outlet
- Requires less bearing-down effort than many other positions
- Relaxes pelvic floor
- May enhance descent if fetus is occiput anterior
- Mechanical advantage: upper trunk presses on fundus more than in other positions
- May enhance woman's sense of security, as she is held closely
- May be awkward for caregiver (who must get on floor to view progress)
- May be tiring for support person who bears woman's weight. If another person is there to help support the woman as in Fig. 6.34, the partner does not become nearly so tired.
- May be less effective if fetus is asynclitic or occiput posterior.

### *When to use lap squatting*

- When second stage progress has arrested
- When woman has joint problems that make squatting impossible
- When woman is too tired to squat or dangle
- When all other positions have been tried.

### *When not to use lap squatting*

- When woman finds it impossible or much more painful
- When there is no strong support person available or woman is too heavy to be supported
- When the woman has an epidural.

## Exaggerated lithotomy (McRoberts' position)

*When:* During second stage.

*How:* The woman lies flat on her back (pillow under her head), legs abducted and knees pulled toward her shoulders (by herself or by two other people, each one drawing one leg up toward one of her shoulders, Fig. 6.35).

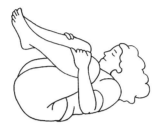

**Fig. 6.35** Exaggerated lithotomy.

### *What this position does*

- Puts fetus in an unfavorable drive angle
- May cause supine hypotension, with resulting reduction in oxygen supply to the fetus
- Is an anti-gravity position
- Is awkward for the woman
- May be beneficial under specific circumstances. If the fetal head is 'stuck' and cannot pass beneath the pubic arch with the woman in other positions, exaggerated lithotomy may help. Pulling the woman's knees toward her shoulders rotates her pelvis posteriorly, flattening the low back and moving her pubic arch up (toward the woman's head)[8,9]. This may allow the fetus to slip under the arch and continue its descent (Fig. 6.36).

6

*Precaution:* If the woman has an epidural, there is danger of injuring her pubic symphysis or sacro-iliac joints by forcing her legs back beyond safe limits. Without sensation, the woman cannot feel the joint pain that would otherwise signal impending damage. Those supporting her legs should resist the temptation to force her legs back, as they could cause serious long-term damage.

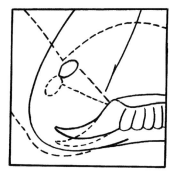

**Fig. 6.36** Exaggerated lithotomy (detail).

### *When to use exaggerated lithotomy*

- When gravity positions and positions to enlarge pelvic diameters have been tried, but the fetus remains 'stuck' at the pubis
- Before forceps or vacuum extraction are used.

### *When not to use exaggerated lithotomy*

- When other, less stressful positions have not been tried first.

## Supine

*When:* During first and second stages.
*How:* The woman lies flat on her back or with her trunk slightly raised (less than 45°). Her legs may be out straight, bent with her feet flat on the bed, in leg rests, or drawn up and back toward her shoulders (Figs 6.37, 6.38).

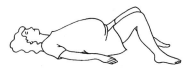

**Fig. 6.37** Supine with knees bent.

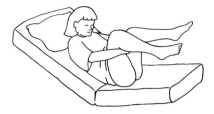

**Fig. 6.38** Supine, head of bed somewhat elevated.

### What this position does

- Allows easy access for vaginal exams
- Allows access if instruments are needed for delivery
- May cause 'supine hypotension' in woman, with resulting reduction in oxygen to the fetus
- May lead to illusion of cephalo-pelvic disproportion due to the reduced pelvic diameters characteristic of this position (often corrected by changing positions)
- Impedes rotation from occiput posterior or occiput transverse to occiput anterior
- Requires woman to push against gravity
- Places fetus in an unfavorable drive angle in relation to pelvis
- Causes contractions to become more frequent, more painful, but less effective than when the woman is vertical.

### When to use the supine position

- When necessary for medical interventions that cannot be done with woman in another position.

### When not to use the supine position

- When medical interventions are not needed.

## MATERNAL MOVEMENTS

This section contains descriptions of movements which may:

- help resolve a fetal malposition such as occiput posterior, persistent occiput transverse, or asynclitism

- enhance fetal descent by altering the shape and size of the woman's pelvic basin
- reduce labor pain, so that the woman is better able to cope with the hours of contractions needed to dilate her cervix and press her fetus through her pelvis
- increase the woman's active participation and decrease her emotional distress, contributing to fetal well-being (see pages 11–16, 179–82)

For information on how to monitor the fetal heart and contractions when women are moving around, see pages 18–25.

### Pelvic rocking (also called pelvic tilt) and other movements of the pelvis

***When:*** Primarily first stage, but also second stage if desired.

***How:*** On hands and knees, the woman 'tucks her seat under' by contracting her abdominal muscles and arching her back, and then relaxes, returning her back to a neutral position (Figs 6.39, 6.40). This is done slowly and rhythmically throughout contractions when she has back pain and presumed OP.

It will be easier on her arms and wrists if she does not bear her weight on her hands but rests her upper body on a support, such as a bean bag, chair, birth ball, or birth bed (Figs 6.41, 6.42).

Other pelvic movements, such as swaying hips from side to side are also helpful. The birth ball allows the woman to roll her upper body on the ball – forward and back, side to side and in circles almost effortlessly.

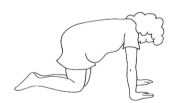

**Fig. 6.39**   Pelvic rocking.

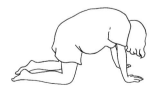

**Fig. 6.40**   Pelvic rocking.

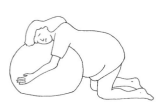

**Fig. 6.41**   Kneeling with birth ball.

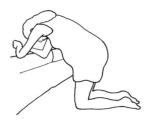

**Fig. 6.42**   Kneeling by a couch.

### *Why pelvic rocking helps*

- If the woman adopts a hands and knees position, gravity encourages rotation of the fetus from OP to OA. The pelvic rocking movement around the fetal head helps to dislodge the head to enable rotation to OA[3].
- The position and movement reduce back pain, by easing pressure of the fetal occiput on the woman's sacro-iliac joint. For many women, this position is the only one they can tolerate when back pain is severe.

### *Advantages*

- Gravity plus movement helps alter the position of the fetus's head within the pelvis, and encourages rotation from OP.
- Relieves back pain.
- If the presumption of OP is in error, this exercise does no harm.

### *Disadvantages*

- The woman's knees may become tired or sore. Knee pads help.
- The belts of the monitor may slip. A support person or caregiver may have to hold the transducer in place (Fig. 6.43), or monitor intermittently. With some monitors it is possible to insert a washcloth between the belt and the transducer (Fig. 6.44), pushing the transducer more snugly against the abdomen to keep it from slipping.

**6**

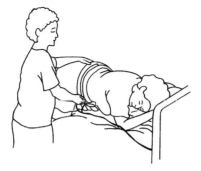

**Fig. 6.43**  Partner holding monitor in place.

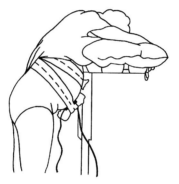

**Fig. 6.44**  Washcloth pressing monitor in place.

## The lunge

**6**

***When:*** Primarily first stage, but also second stage if desired.

***How***: Stabilize a chair so that it will not slide. The woman stands, facing forward with the chair at her side. She raises one foot, places it on the chair seat, and rotates her raised knee and foot to a right angle from the direction in which she is facing (Fig. 6.45). Keeping her body upright, she shifts her weight sideways (lunges), bending her raised knee. She remains in that position for a few seconds, then returns to upright. She repeats this throughout several contractions in a row. She should feel a stretch in both inner thighs; if not, she should widen the distance between the foot on the floor and the foot on the chair. Her partner helps her with balance.

The lunge can also be done on a bed in the kneeling position. See Fig. 6.46.

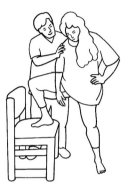
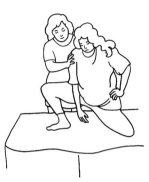

**Fig. 6.45**   Standing lunge.          **Fig. 6.46**   Kneeling lunge.

### *Deciding which direction to lunge*

If the baby is OP, the woman should lunge in the direction of the occiput (e.g. if the fetus is LOP, she lunges to the left). Lunging to this side probably feels better.

Even if the baby is not known to be OP and the woman has no back pain, the lunge may be useful at any time when active labor progress has slowed. The changes in pelvic shape caused by the lunge may correct subtle fetal positional problems. The woman will probably find that lunging to one side feels better than the other. The side that feels better is probably the one that gives more room for the occiput to adjust.

**6**

### *Why the lunge helps*

The elevated femur acts as a lever at the hip joint, 'prying' one ischium outward. This creates more space in that side of the pelvis for the posterior occiput to rotate, or the asynclitic occiput to resolve its position. Lunging also uses gravity to advantage.

### *Advantages*

- Facilitates rotation
- Reduces back pain
- Allows the partner to provide physical and emotional support.

### *Disadvantages*

- The woman should have someone (partner, doula or caregiver) close by to help her maintain her balance
- The woman with joint problems in her legs or hips should not do the lunge.

## Walking or stair climbing

*When:* Primarily first stage, but also second stage if desired.
*How:* The woman walks or climbs stairs (Figs 6.47, 6.48), continuing during contractions if possible. If not, she leans on her partner or the banister. If she spreads her feet wide apart on each stair, in effect she is 'lunging' and climbing stairs at the same time.

### *Why walking and stair climbing help*

Slight but repeated changes in the alignment of pelvic joints occur with each step (more so with stair climbing), encouraging fetal rotation and descent. Walking and stair climbing also use gravity to advantage.

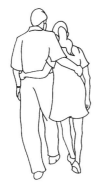

**Fig. 6.47**  Walking.

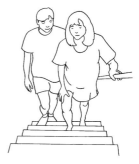

**Fig. 6.48**  Stair climbing.

### Advantages

- Facilitates fetal rotation
- Often improves morale, especially if it provides a change of scene.

### Disadvantages

- May be tiring
- Stairs may be inconveniently located.

## Slow dancing

***When:*** Primarily first stage, but also second stage, if desired.

***How:*** The woman stands and leans on partner, and sways slowly from side to side. They stand facing each other, with partner embracing woman and pressing on her low back. She leans on him, with her arms relaxed at her sides or with her thumbs hooked into her partner's back pockets or waistband. She rests her head on her partner's shoulder or chest. They can sway to their favorite music and she can breathe in the rhythm of the 'dance'. This is the most relaxing and least tiring way to maintain a standing position, since the woman is partially supported (Fig. 6.49).

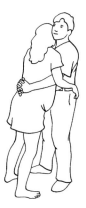

**Fig. 6.49**  Slow dancing.

### Why slow dancing helps

Slight but repeated changes in the pelvic joints occur as she sways, encouraging fetal rotation and descent. The vertical position uses gravity to advantage.

### Advantages

- Partner's embrace and support may reduce her emotional stress and her catecholamine production, enabling her uterus to work more efficiently.
- The partner provides a kind of support that no one else can give as well. For partners who want to help but feel at a loss to know how, it is most gratifying
- Rhythmic swaying movements are comforting, and may enable her to relax her trunk and pelvic muscles
- Partner can press on woman's lower back, providing counter-pressure to relieve back pain
- Can be done beside the bed, with monitors and intravenous lines attached to her body
- Good substitute for walking.

### Disadvantages

- Woman needs a partner with whom she feels comfortable 'slow dancing'.
- Height discrepancies between woman and partner may make slow dancing uncomfortable or impossible.

Similar physical benefits can be gained if the woman leans and sways over a birth ball placed on a table or birth bed. She can also lean and sway on the bed, counter, or wall.

## Abdominal stroking

*When:* Primarily first stage, but also second stage if desired.
*How:* The woman gets into a hands-and-knees position. Her caregiver or partner stands beside her on the side opposite the fetal occiput. The helper reaches beneath the woman's abdomen and, placing one hand on the woman's side, firmly and smoothly strokes across

the woman's abdomen, toward the helper (in the direction toward which the occiput should rotate). For example, if the fetus is ROP, the helper stands on the woman's left side, reaches beneath her abdomen to her right side and strokes her abdomen toward the left. The stroking stops at about the middle of the woman's abdomen. See Fig. 6.50.

The stroking movement is done between contractions, and is rhythmic in character. The stroke should be firm enough to lift the abdomen slightly; this usually feels very good to the woman.

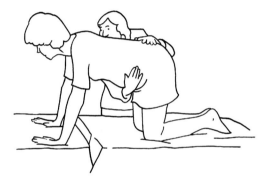

**Fig. 6.50**    Abdominal stroking for an LOP fetus.

### *Why abdominal stroking helps*

Use abdominal stroking to help turn an OP baby *if* the position (LOP or ROP) is known. With gravity and external stroking of the abdomen in the direction the baby needs to rotate, the likelihood is increased that the baby will rotate[2].

### *When to use abdominal stroking*

- Whenever the fetus is clearly in an OP position, and the direction of the occiput is known
- Can be used before labor or during early labor. Success is more likely if the head is unengaged.

**6**

### *When not to use abdominal stroking*

- When fetal position is not known
- When the woman is unable to get into or remain in the hands-and-knees position.

## Abdominal lifting

***When:*** Primarily first stage, but also second stage if desired.

***How:*** The woman stands upright. During the contraction she interlocks the fingers of both hands beneath her abdomen and lifts her abdomen upward and inward, while bending her knees to tilt her pelvis[10] (Fig. 6.51). She maintains the lift throughout the contraction. Her partner (depending on her size and the length of the partner's arms) may be able to assist with abdominal lifting by standing behind the woman and reaching around to lift her abdomen.

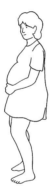

**Fig. 6.51** Abdominal lifting.

### *Why abdominal lifting helps*

Abdominal lifting can help align the long axis of the fetus with the axis of the pelvic inlet. This improves fetal positioning and the efficiency of contractions. Abdominal lifting is particularly helpful for those women with:

- back pain in labor associated with a fetal occiput posterior position
- or such maternal conditions as:

- ○ a pronounced swayback
- ○ pendulous abdomen (weak abdominal muscles)
- ○ a short waist (from iliac crests to lowest ribs)
- ○ some previous low back injuries.

### *Advantages*

- Reduces back pain
- Provides gravity advantage
- May be done at any stage of labor, from pre-labor into the second stage
- Sometimes leads to rapid labor (especially in multiparas with pendulous abdomens).

### *Disadvantages*

- Is tiring for the woman if done over a long period
- Since rapid progress sometimes occurs suddenly, this should not be done with strong active labor contractions until woman is where she intends to give birth.

## The pelvic press

***When:*** Second stage.

***How:*** With the woman in a squatting position, the partner or caregiver kneels behind her, and during a contraction locates her iliac crests and presses them very firmly toward each other (Fig. 6.52). This should cause some movement in the pelvis, which slightly narrows the upper pelvis. The ilia pivot at the sacro-iliac joints, causing the mid-pelvis and the pelvic outlet to widen. Combining the pelvic press with the squatting position will give the greatest chance of increasing space within the pelvis. Within three or four contractions, there should be some evidence of rotation or descent[11].

**6**

### *How the pelvic press helps*

The pelvic press is a technique for enlarging the midpelvic and inter-tuberous diameters in second stage. The added room may allow rotation and descent in cases of a malposition or 'tight fit' at the pelvic outlet.

(a)

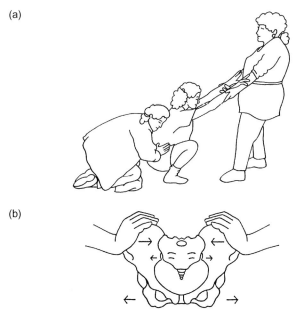

(b)

**Fig. 6.52**   (a) Pelvic press. (b) Pelvic press (detail).

### *When to use the pelvic press*

- In second stage, when there is a delay in descent or a caput forming (due to malposition or cephalo-pelvic disproportion)
- In second stage, when a woman reports severe back pain.

### *When not to use the pelvic press*

- When the pelvic press causes severe bone or joint pain, as it might if the woman has arthritis or a previous injury to her pelvis
- When the woman has an epidural, because without sensation, joints could be damaged.

## Other rhythmic movements

***When:*** First or second stage.
***How:*** Moving their bodies rhythmically often seems to occur

instinctively in women who are coping well in labor. Rocking in a chair (Fig. 6.53), or swaying while sitting on a birth ball (Fig. 6.54) or while standing and leaning over a tray table (Fig. 6.55) or birth ball that is placed on a bed (Fig. 6.56), are examples of such rhythmic bodily movements. If a woman with slow labor progress is not spontaneously moving as described here, the caregiver might suggest that she try it.

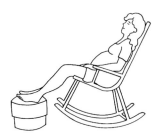

**Fig. 6.53**  Sitting in a rocking chair.

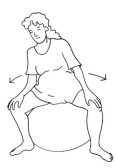

**Fig. 6.54**  Sitting, swaying on a birth ball.

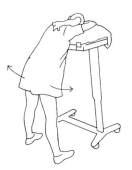

**Fig. 6.55**  Standing, swaying with a tray table.

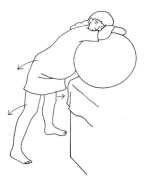

**Fig. 6.56**  Standing, swaying with a ball.

6

### *Why rhythmic movements help*

- Rhythmic movements tend to be calming
- Rhythmic movements may alter the relationships among fetus, pelvis, and gravity to promote progress.

When spontaneous, rocking is often an indication that the woman is coping well.

## REFERENCES

1. Roberts, J. (1989) Maternal positions during the first stage of labour. In: *Effective Care in Pregnancy and Childbirth*, vol. 2. Chalmers, I., Enkin, M., Keirse, M.J.N.C. (eds). Oxford University Press, Oxford.
2. Enkin, M., Keirse, M.J.N.C., Renfrew, M. and Neilson, J. (1995) *A Guide to Effective Care in Pregnancy and Childbirth*. Oxford University Press, Oxford.
3. Andrews, C. and Andrews, E. (1983) Nursing, maternal postures, and fetal position. *Nurs. Res.* **32** (6), 336–41.
4. Hofmeyr, G.J. (1998) Hands/knees posture in late pregnancy or labour for malposition (lateral or posterior) of the presenting part. (Cochrane Review). In the Cochrane Library (database on disk and CD-ROM), Issue 2, Updated quarterly. The Cochrane Collaboration. Update Software, Oxford.
5. Sutton, J. and Scott, P. (1996) *Understanding and Teaching Optimal Foetal Positioning*. Birth Concepts, Tauranga, NZ.
6. Fenwick, L. and Simkin, P. (1987) Maternal positioning to prevent or alleviate dystocia in labor. *Clin. Obstet. Gynecol.* **30(1)**, 83–9.
7. El Halta, V. (1995) Posterior labor: A pain in the back. *Midwif. Today* **36**, 19–21.
8. Smeltzer, J.S. (1986) Prevention and management of shoulder dystocia. *Clin. Obstet. Gynecol.* **29(2)**, 299–308.
9. Sweet, B.R. and Tiran, D. (eds) (1997) *Mayes' Midwifery*. Baillière Tindall, London.
10. King, J.M. (1993) *Back Labor No More!!!* Plenary System, Dallas.
11. Koehler, N. (1985) *Artemis Speaks: VBAC Stories and Natural Childbirth Information*. Jerald R. Brown, Occidental, California.

**6**

Chapter 7

# The Labor Progress Toolkit: Part 2. Comfort Measures

*Note:* Please see Chapters 2 and 6 for general measures to aid labor progress.

In cases of dystocia, there is another important goal besides improving labor progress. That is to help the woman keep her pain within manageable limits, if possible, without interfering with her ability to

7

move freely. This can sometimes be accomplished by using the non-pharmacological pain relief measures described in this section.

We do want to acknowledge the benefits of a well timed epidural in serious cases of dystocia: as a precursor to painful interventions; as an aid for an exhausted mother to get some sleep; and possibly to create, in effect, a 'mind–body split' in cases where deep-seated fear or anxiety is an underlying cause of dystocia. We hope this book will help prevent dystocia from becoming arrested labor, which often necessitates profound pain relief for a good outcome.

Following are general comfort guidelines for slow labors:

- Frequent position changes (about every 20 to 30 minutes when progress is slow) shorten labor, and may reduce the woman's pain significantly. See Chapter 6 for information on specific positions. When progress is adequate, there is no need to change anything.

- Rhythmic movement reduces both pain and anxiety. See Chapter 6, page 151 for more information on why movement helps and specific movements to try. For information on monitoring the mobile woman's fetus, see Chapter 2, pages 18–25.

- Pressure techniques as shown on pages 182–6 reduce back pain.

- Heat and cold as shown later in this chapter (pages 167–70) reduce various types of pain.

- Hydrotherapy as shown on pages 170–74 reduces muscle tension, pain and anxiety dramatically for many women. Immersion in water also provides buoyancy (reducing the effect of gravity on the woman, not on the fetus), even distribution of hydrostatic pressure over the immersed parts of the woman's body, and warmth, often resulting in pain relief and more rapid progress in active labor.

- Techniques such as relaxation, naturalistic breathing patterns and bearing-down efforts give many women a sense of mastery over their pain and help them get through a long, potentially worrisome labor. See pages 195–8 for suggestions on the use of such techniques.

- Continuous labor support by a trained, experienced doula, or professional labor support person helps the woman or couple with emotional support, physical comfort, non-clinical advice, and assistance in getting information.

The use of doulas is increasing, especially in North America, as scientific evidence of their benefit builds[1,2]. In settings where midwives and nurses can spend time with women or couples in a non-clinical capacity, similar benefits can be achieved by professional caregivers. See page 176 for information on continuous support and doula care.

## NON-PHARMACOLOGICAL PHYSICAL COMFORT MEASURES

### Heat

***How:***

- Apply a hot moist towel, heating pad, heated silica gel pack, heated rice pack or hot water bottle to lower abdomen, groin, thighs, lower back, shoulders, or perineum, or
- Direct a warm shower on her shoulders, abdomen, or lower back, or suggest she immerse herself in warm water. (See Hydrotherapy, page 170) or
- Apply warmed blanket to her entire body.

*Caution:* Compresses should not be uncomfortably hot to the person applying them. Women in labor may have an altered perception of temperature and may not react to excessive heat even if it is causing a burn. Wrap one or two (or more) layers of towelling, or a plastic disposable bed pad around the source of heat as needed to ensure it is not too hot. Put nothing on the woman's skin that you cannot hold in your hand.

#### *How heat helps*

Heat (Fig. 7.1) increases local skin temperature, circulation, and tissue metabolism. It reduces muscle spasm and raises the pain threshold. Heat also reduces the 'fight or flight' response (as evidenced by trembling and 'goose pimples')[3]. Local heat or a warm blanket calms the woman, and also may increase her receptivity to a stroking type of massage which she cannot tolerate when her skin is sensitive or sore due to the fight or flight response.

One small study of heat (a hot water bottle) applied to the fundus found that it increased uterine activity[4].

7

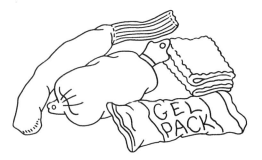

**Fig. 7.1** Heat.

*Please note:* Rice-filled microwaveable packs can be purchased in many department stores. Or they can easily be made by the woman by filling a man's tube sock with $1\frac{1}{2}$ pounds (0.68 kg) of dry uncooked rice and stitching the top of the sock closed. Three to five minutes in a microwave oven set on High, or 10 minutes in a ceramic dish in a 180°F oven provides moist heat for up to half an hour. Adding lavender seeds or flowers to the rice makes for a lovely aroma. Rice packs can be reheated for the same woman, but should not be reused by other clients. *Caution:* If the rice pack is being reheated in a microwave oven that is also used to heat food, caution should be exercised to avoid contaminating the oven with the woman's body fluids. Place the rice pack in a glass or plastic container or consult your infection control department if this is a concern. (Rice packs can also be frozen to use as cold packs.)

*A further caution:* Never place any hot object on a laboring woman if it cannot be held in one's hands without discomfort.

### When to use heat

- When the woman reports or shows pain in a specific area
- When the woman reports or shows signs of anxiety or muscle tension
- When the woman reports feeling chilled
- When increased uterine activity is desirable. (Put warm compress or hot water bottle on abdomen over fundus.)
- In the second stage, hot compresses on the perineum enhance relaxation of the pelvic floor and reduce pain.

### When not to use heat

- When the woman reports feeling uncomfortably warm or has a fever
- If staff are worried about potential harm from the heat.

## Cold

### How:

- Apply cold compresses to lower back, or perineum, using an ice bag, gel pack, rice pack, latex glove filled with ice chips, frozen wet wash cloth, cold can of soft drink, plastic bottle of frozen water, or another cold object (Fig. 7.2a)
- Provide a large strap-on gel pack (available from sports medicine suppliers) to the low back. This allows the woman to move or walk around (Fig. 7.2b)
- Use a cold moist wash cloth to cool a sweating woman's face, hands, or arms
- Place a frozen gel pack or plastic bottle of frozen water against the anus to relieve painful hemorrhoids in second stage

Always put one or two layers of fabric or a disposable bed pad between the cold item and the woman's skin. This avoids the sudden discomfort that would occur with the direct application of cold to the skin, and allows for a gradual and well-tolerated shift from feeling cool to feeling cold.

### How cold helps

Cold is especially useful for musculoskeletal and joint pain. Cold decreases muscle spasm (for longer than heat). It numbs the area by slowing the transmission of pain and other impulses over sensory neurons (which helps to explain the often noted numbing effects of cold). Cold also reduces swelling and is cooling to the skin[3].

### When to use cold

- When woman reports back pain in labor
- When woman feels overheated or is sweating during labor
- When hemorrhoids cause excessive pain
- After the birth, as a cold compress on the woman's perineum to relieve swelling or stitch pain.

**7**

(a)                                    (b)

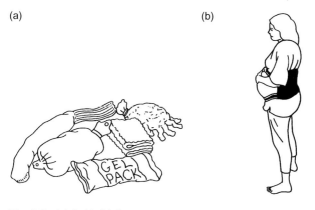

**Fig. 7.2**   (a) Cold. (b) Strap-on cold-pack.

### When not to use

- When woman is already feeling chilled. Use heat first in this case
- For women from cultures in which the use of cold is a threat to the woman's well being during labor or postpartum. Ask her if she prefers a hot pack or a cold pack or nothing
- When the woman reports that the use of cold is not helping her or is irritating.

## Hydrotherapy

***How:*** Have woman stand or sit on a stool in the shower (Fig. 7.3). A bath that allows deep water and room for the partner and for the woman to move around seems most beneficial and is most popular (Fig. 7.4). *Caution:* Water temperature in the bath should not exceed 98–100°F or 37–37.5°C, because warmer water may raise the woman's temperature and cause fetal tachycardia.

### How hydrotherapy helps

Hydrotherapy reduces muscle tension, pain and anxiety dramatically for many women. Immersion in water also provides buoyancy (reducing the effect of gravity on the woman, not on the fetus), even distribution of hydrostatic pressure over the immersed portions of the

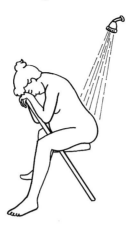

**Fig. 7.3** Shower.

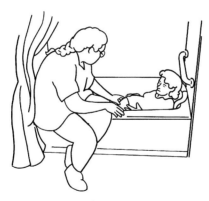

**Fig. 7.4** Bath.

woman's body, and warmth, all of which often bring pain relief and more rapid active labor progress.

### *How to monitor the fetus in or around water:*

- Hand-held Doppler device: the woman lifts her abdomen out of the water or steps out of the shower for intermittent monitoring.

7

- Waterproof hand-held Doppler used in bath or shower (Fig. 7.5a).
- Standard electronic fetal monitoring tocodynamometers and ultrasound transducers ('belt monitors') are used with telemetry units underwater in some hospitals with women who must be monitored continuously (Fig. 7.5b). The sensors are highly water resistant and the battery-powered units operate on very low voltage, so these hospitals consider them safe to the woman and fetus. The sensors are usually covered with waterproof gloves or long plastic bags that also cover the wires. These covers are used more to protect the equipment than the woman[5]. (*Please note:* Before trying

(a)

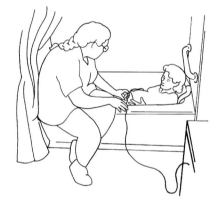

(b)

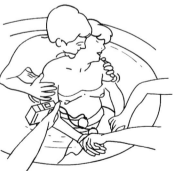

**Fig. 7.5**   (a) Monitoring in bath. (b) Telemetry in bath.

this, however, contact your hospital's biomedical services or engineering department regarding both safety and any potential equipment damage connected with using the tocodynamometer and ultrasound device under water.)

### When to use hydrotherapy

- As a possible alternative to bedrest for women with pregnancy induced hypertension[6].
- *Showers:* Use in any phase of first stage labor or early second stage.
- *Immersion in bath:* Use after active labor is established. Because immersion in water often slows contractions if used before active labor, a bath is sometimes recommended to stop pre-term contractions or to slow exhausting pre-labor contractions to give the woman some temporary rest. Entrance into the water before 5 cm, however, has been associated with longer labor and greater need for oxytocin augmentation[7].

*Note 1:* Immersion in deep water when one is in pre-term labor, pre-labor, or latent labor often stops contractions temporarily. The hydrostatic pressure (the weight of the water) moves tissue fluid into the intravascular space, increasing plasma volume[6]. This may dilute circulating oxytocin or prostaglandins, which could slow or temporarily stop early labor. By the time active labor is established, however, these effects are less pronounced and seem to be overshadowed by the relaxing and pain-relieving effects of the water. Often active labor dilation speeds up when the woman enters the bath[7].

*Note 2:* No significant adverse effects have been reported from immersion in water in labor, such as maternal and newborn infection, or other newborn outcomes, but 'the use of water immersion during labour should be encouraged only with caution until more evidence to determine the safety of immersion on the fetus and newborn is available'[8].

### When not to use hydrotherapy

### Showers:
- When the woman's balance or ability to stand is unreliable, due to medication or other reasons

7

- When there is a medical contraindication requiring restriction to bed.

### *Immersion in a bath:*
- Before active labor is established (unless slowing of labor or temporary cessation of contractions is desired)
- When there is a medical contraindication such as bleeding or fetal distress
- When birth is imminent (unless woman and practitioner are planning a water birth)
- When the woman has received medications or an epidural for pain.

### *Effectiveness of hydrotherapy*

A recent meta-analysis of the trials of immersion in water during labor found no clear benefits, or risks[8]. However, when one examines trials that investigated the timing (in terms of dilation) of entry into the bath[7], or investigated effects only of a late bath compared with no bath[9], the results indicate benefits in terms of labor progress and pain reduction in women who used the bath after 5 cm. In randomized trials of immersion in water during active labor compared with either no bath or early bath, the following findings have been reported:

- Cervices changed more rapidly (Bishop scores) in the late bath group[9].
- Pain increased more slowly in the bath group[9].
- Labor augmentation was required half as often in the late bath group compared with the early bath group[7].

Patient satisfaction with hydrotherapy seems to be high[10], which makes it very important to study its potential benefits and risks, and to discover the safest and most beneficial methods for its use.

Showers have not been studied systematically, but clinical experience suggests many women experience enhanced maternal relaxation, and significant reductions in pain.

## Acupressure

*How:* Pressure on the points illustrated in Fig. 7.6 during labor is thought to enhance contractions without increasing labor pain.

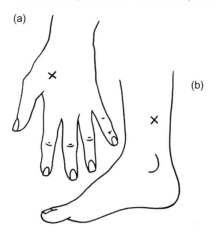

**Fig. 7.6** Ho-ku point on hand (on the back of the hand where the metacarpal bones of the thumb and the index finger come together); Spleen 6 point on ankle (on the tibia, four finger widths above the medial malleolus (inner ankle bone): press in on the tibia and diagonally forward; this point will be very tender).

(1) Press firmly with a finger on the point for 10–60 seconds. Then rest for an equal length of time.
(2) Repeat this cycle for up to six cycles. Contractions should speed up during that time.

### *How acupressure helps*

Acupressure is based on acupuncture theory, which states that specific health problems, including poor progress or excessive pain in labor, arise when there is a blockage of energy flow along particular meridians in the body. By releasing the blockage, harmony and smooth functioning return. Acupressure has never been subjected to scientific evaluation, so its effectiveness is not certain[11]. However, the techniques are simple and, when used as described here, appear free of harmful effects. They may therefore be worth trying when contractions are excessively painful and labor progress is inadequate.

7

### When to use acupressure

- When labor induction is considered necessary. The woman might try self-help measures to start labor, in hopes of avoiding induction, but only after discussing this with her doctor or midwife
- In labor, when more frequent contractions are desired or needed
- When contractions are very painful but not accompanied by labor progress.

### When not to use acupressure

- During pregnancy before term (unless induction is being planned), because it may result in pre-term labor contractions. We also suggest that the woman not even experiment with it on herself before labor
- If she has not consulted her doctor or midwife.

## Continuous labor support from a doula, nurse, or midwife

Until recently, and even today, nurses and midwives, along with women's partners, have been designated as the people to provide support to laboring women. Professional staff were expected to add labor support to their long list of other tasks, and it was assumed that any knowledgeable professional could easily do this without instruction. The partner was assumed to be calm and capable enough to 'coach' a woman through labor. But recently, the emergence of the doula has shown that labor support cannot be an 'add-on' to other duties, nor can a loved one provide all the support a woman needs[12,13]. We now realize that labor support deserves more emphasis than it has received.

A *doula* is a person (usually a woman), trained and experienced in childbirth, who accompanies laboring women and their partners throughout labor and birth (Figs 7.7a, b). She provides continuous emotional support, physical comfort, and non-clinical advice. She is usually a lay person, although some nurses and childbirth educators have become doulas.

(a)

(b)

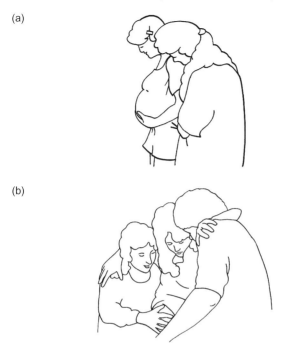

**Fig. 7.7**  (a) Doula supporting a woman. (b) Doula supporting a couple.

### How the doula helps

The doula focuses on the woman through each contraction, offering reassurance, praise, encouragement, and comfort, and she also instructs and reassures the woman's partner. She rarely takes a break and remains with the woman until after the birth. Doulas usually do not work shifts. The doula performs no clinical tasks. Her sole responsibility is the woman's and the partner's emotional well-being and the woman's physical comfort. Some hospitals and health agencies have doulas on staff to help women as they are admitted, but most doulas contract privately with clients. Some work as volunteers; most charge a fee.

In North America, doulas are certified by Doulas of North America (DONA), the International Childbirth Education Association (ICEA), and the Association of Labor Assistants and Childbirth Educators (ALACE). The concept of the doula is newer in the UK and Europe.

### When to use a doula

A doula should be used whenever one is available and the woman wants her services. There are no known harmful effects when doulas, as described above, are in attendance.

### When not to use a doula

A doula should not be used when the woman or her partner prefers not to have one.

### Effectiveness of doulas

Eleven randomized controlled studies[1,2] have shown that women who are accompanied by experienced doulas during labor have:

- shorter labors
- less need for oxytocin augmentation in labor
- fewer operative vaginal deliveries
- fewer cesareans
- fewer requests for pain medication
- fewer newborns with Apgar scores < 7
- greater patient satisfaction
- more positive maternal–infant interactions two months later[14]
- less postpartum depression 6 weeks after birth[15].

### What about staff nurses and midwives as labor support providers?

'There are two common barriers to be overcome before nurses can provide skilled labor support to their patients: lack of time and lack of knowledge'[16].

While many maternity nurses and midwives enjoy and are skilled in the labor support role, others have little knowledge of these skills since labor support does not hold a high priority in most educational programs. One recent study reported a wide variation in the cesarean section rates among the patients of individual nurses in one large hospital[17]. A major difference between the nurses with the lowest and highest cesarean rates was that the nurses with the lowest rates took greater interest in each woman's psychosocial history and circumstances. This may indicate that they were more concerned with the emotional needs of their laboring patients.

However, even the most knowledgeable and supportive nurse cannot always provide the continuous care that contributes to improved obstetric outcomes, especially if she is responsible for more than one laboring woman or must assume other clinical or 'indirect' patient care tasks that take her out of the woman's room.

What about midwives? Continuous one-to-one care by midwives who focus on psychosocial aspects of childbirth has been shown to produce more favorable outcomes when compared with the usual care by obstetricians[18]. In North America, though numbers are increasing, there are still relatively few midwives or doulas, and nurses tend to be very busy with multiple tasks, all of which leaves many laboring women with little professional support. One can only speculate about the contribution of a lack of emotional support to the incidence of labor dystocia.

## PSYCHOSOCIAL COMFORT MEASURES

In Chapter 2 we discussed the importance of a peaceful environment for birth, and showed how outside disturbances may interfere with the labor process. We also described the labor-inhibiting effects of disturbance, fear and anxiety, and how excessive production of stress hormones (catecholamines) can affect uterine and placental function. Chapter 2 also listed some basic and universal guidelines for helping women adapt to the labor environment, and for adapting the labor environment to each woman.

In Chapter 6 and the previous section of this chapter, we provided many physical measures to improve comfort and progress.

This section presents specific psychosocial comfort measures that calm the laboring woman's distress and enhance her feelings of emotional safety.

### Assessing the woman's emotional state

It is not always possible to assess a woman's sense of well-being by observation. A woman who is still and quiet during contractions may actually be feeling as though she is 'screaming inside,' or 'barely keeping the lid on.' Another woman who is vocal and active may feel okay as long as she can express and release her feelings, or, as one

7

woman said, 'shout the pain down.' A woman's external façade is not always an accurate reflection of how she really feels. Sometimes the best way to assess her well-being is to ask her.

To assess the woman's emotional state, it often helps to ask the woman, between contractions, 'What was going through your mind during that contraction?' Her answer may tell much about her emotional needs, and about whether she is coping well or is distressed. This knowledge will help those around her to provide appropriate emotional support. One important study found that if a woman has distressing thoughts during latent phase contractions (possibly indicating excessive catecholamine production), she is at increased risk for prolonged labor, fetal distress, and all the interventions that accompany such problems. This was not true when women's distressing thoughts occurred in active labor. 'We conclude that latent labor is a critical phase in the psychobiology of labor and that pain and cognitive activity (thoughts) during this phase are important contributions to labor efficiency and obstetric outcome'[19].

Therefore, elimination or reduction of stress is a worthwhile goal, especially in early labor when a woman has little need for clinical care.

Following are specific ways to reduce stress and enhance the woman's emotional well-being.

*Provide reassuring or comforting sensory stimuli:*

- music that the woman likes
- hand massage, back rub
- lighting that suits the woman
- juice or frozen juice bars in a flavor she likes
- pleasant-smelling hand cream or massage oil
- make electronic fetal monitoring heart tones audible if the woman finds them reassuring; otherwise, turn them down.

*Provide reassurance and praise:*

- Ask what sensations the woman is feeling. Explain what causes them and reassure her that these sensations are normal. 'Your body knows just what it's doing'; 'I know this is difficult. It's because you're making good progress. It won't be much longer.'
- Suggest comfort measures to her and her partner.
- Compliment her: 'You're doing so well'; 'Don't change a thing'; 'You're perfect.'

- Explain monitor tracings to the woman if they are reassuring. Respect her wishes regarding information if they are not reassuring.
- Mention to a colleague, within the woman's hearing, something that is going well about the woman's labor, or something she is doing particularly well.
- Explain that the noisy woman next door says it helps her cope or push when she yells. And, if culturally appropriate, you might add, 'You might also find that helpful at some point.'
- Help her reframe distressing thoughts, especially in early labor: 'Can you imagine your strong contractions doing exactly what they are supposed to do – open your cervix and bring your baby to you?'

*Reduce fear-inducing stimuli and actions:*

- Close the woman's door and that of any vocal women.
- Minimize interventions if the woman does not want them (especially painful or invasive ones).
- Turn down the volume on EFM if the woman does not like it.
- Ask other staff to make sure they cannot possibly be overheard when discussing their patients. Information and vocabulary that are emotionally neutral to staff members may be frightening to the woman.
- If the woman is accompanied by someone who makes her anxious, ask her privately if she would like that person to leave the room. (Send him or her on an errand, suggest they get a snack.) If necessary, ask that person to wait elsewhere.
- Children at birth should be accompanied by their own support people, so the woman and her support person(s) can focus on coping with the labor.
- Avoid bringing unnecessary staff members into the woman's room.

*Provide a more private, less inhibiting environment:*

- Remember that nudity or being scantily clad is threatening or embarrassing for some people. Offer an extra gown or robe to cover the woman's back. Some women feel more like themselves if they wear their own clothing in labor, while some want no clothes on.
- Keep curtain and/or door closed.
- Knock before entering and encourage other staff to do the same.
- Encourage the anxious woman to spend some time in the bathroom

7

with the door closed. Sometimes women need privacy, a small space, and freedom from disturbances to adjust psychologically to the demands of labor. Labor progress sometimes improves after some private time. Many women who are 'holding back' can relax their pelvic floors on the toilet. If you are concerned that the baby may be born suddenly, instruct the woman to push the call light in the bathroom if she feels a lot of pressure.

- Encourage and reinforce the woman's spontaneous coping behaviors, such as rhythmic movements, sounds, and position changes. ('You are good at finding the positions and sounds that work for you.')
- If you are not sure whether a specific behavior is helping the woman or is simply a sign of distress, ask non-judgementally. ('Does it help to shake your hands during the contraction?')
- Encourage the use of hydrotherapy. Many women 'let go' in the shower or bath.

For ways to support women in pre-labor and latent first stage, see pages 34–7. For information on emotional dystocia in active first stage labor, see pages 70–75. See pages 119–21 for information on emotional dystocia and 'holding back' in second stage labor.

## TECHNIQUES AND DEVICES TO REDUCE BACK PAIN

### Counterpressure

***How:*** The woman's partner exerts steady pressure throughout the contraction on the woman's sacrum with the heel or fist of one hand (Figs 7.8a, b). The woman tells the partner where to push (wherever the pain is most intense) and how hard.

If needed, the partner places his other hand on the front of the woman's hip (over the anterior superior iliac spine) to help her keep her balance.

#### *How counterpressure helps*

It is not clear exactly how or why counterpressure eases back pain in labor. It may change the shape of the pelvis enough to ease pain caused by the pressure of the posterior occiput on the sacro-iliac joints.

(a)

(b)

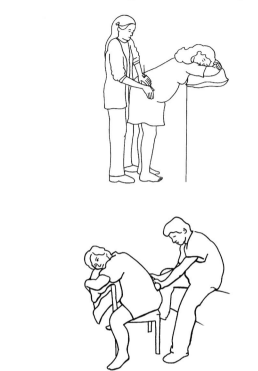

**Fig. 7.8** (a) Counterpressure. (b) Counterpressure with tennis balls.

Judging from its popularity with women, every caregiver should know and be able to teach partners how to do counterpressure.

### When to use counterpressure

- When the woman reports back pain.

### When not to use counterpressure

- When the woman reports counterpressure is not helping, or when she finds it distracting.

7

## The double hip squeeze

***How:*** The partner places his hands on the outsides of the woman's hips, over the woman's gluteal muscles (well below her iliac crests, over the 'meatiest' part of her buttocks) and presses inward toward the center of her pelvis with the whole palms of his hands (not just the heels of his hands) steadily throughout the contraction. The woman decides how much pressure she needs, and exactly where he should place his hands.

*Note:* this is different from the 'pelvic press,' which is used in cases of deep transverse arrest, persistent occiput posterior, or in cases of borderline cephalo-pelvic disproportion. See page 161 for a description.

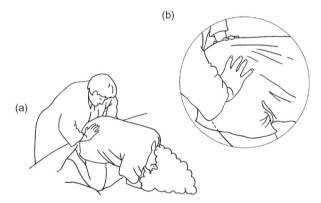

**Fig. 7.9** (a) Double hip squeeze. (b) Double hip squeeze detail.

### How the double hip squeeze helps

It is not clear how or why the double hip squeeze (Figs 7.9a, b) eases back pain in labor. The pressure may change the shape of the pelvis as does counterpressure (see preceding section). It may slightly reduce the stretch in the sacro-iliac joints, easing the strain on those ligaments caused by internal pressure of the malpositioned fetal head.

*Note:* The authors consider it a poor prognosis if a woman needs extreme pressure in the double hip squeeze (i.e. requiring all the strength of her partner) in order to get relief. We believe that such

**7**

extreme measures may indicate that the fetal head is deeply engaged and less likely to rotate spontaneously than when moderate or minor pressure is sufficient to relieve pain. In fact, one may wonder if the extreme pressure would decrease the volume in the pelvic basin and actually impair rotation. This question should be researched: the double hip squeeze seems very effective in relieving pain, but it should not come at the cost of rotation!

Other measures, such as the open knee–chest position (Chapter 6, page 139), abdominal lifting (Chapter 6, page 160), the knee press (page 185), or the use of cold (page 169) or heat (page 167), or the pelvic press in second stage (Chapter 6, page 161) or an epidural may be preferable to maximal pressure in the double hip squeeze.

### When to use the double hip squeeze

- When the woman reports back pain.

### When not to use the double hip squeeze

- When the woman reports that it is not helping.

## The knee press

***How:*** *If the woman is seated:* Woman sits upright on a straight chair with her low back against the back of the chair. She places her feet flat on the floor and her knees a few inches apart. (If her feet do not reach the floor, books or other supports can be placed beneath each foot (Fig. 7.10a).)

Her partner kneels on the floor in front of her and cups his hands over her knees. Locking his elbows in close to his trunk, and rising off his haunches, he leans toward the woman throughout each contraction, allowing his upper body weight to apply pressure on her knees, which is directed from his hands straight back toward her hip joints. She feels a slight release in her low back and relief of back pain.

*If the woman is sidelying, with one or two pillows supporting her upper knee:* Two partners are needed (Fig. 7.10b). Only the upper knee is pressed. The woman bends her upper knee and hip joints to 90° angles. One partner presses on the woman's sacrum during contractions to stabilize her. The other partner cups the woman's top knee in his or her other hand and presses on that knee directly back toward her hip joint.

7

(a)

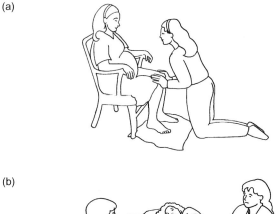

(b)

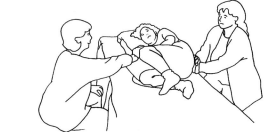

**Fig. 7.10** (a) Knee press – seated. (b) Knee press – lateral.

### *How the knee press helps*

Pressure directed via the femur straight into the flexed hip joint or joints alters the configuration of the pelvic basin, releasing the sacro-iliac joints, and relieving low back pain.

### *When to use the knee press*

- When the woman has back pain.

### *When not to use the knee press*

- When the woman reports the knee press is not reducing her pain
- When the woman has joint pain, inflammation, or damage in her knee joints.

7

## Cold and heat

*Cold and rolling cold:* See page 169, for the rationale and complete instructions; see also Figs 7.11 and 7.12.

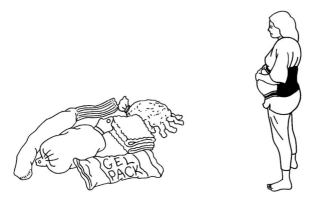

**Fig. 7.11** Cold.    **Fig. 7.12** Strap-on cold-pack.

*Note:* Always enclose the cold object in one or two layers of cloth to protect the woman from the sudden shock of a freezing object directly placed on her skin.

Pressing and rolling a cold can of juice or soft drink over the woman's low back is sometimes appreciated more than steady pressure in one area.

### Hot compresses

See page 167 for more information.

*Note:* The woman's temperature sense may be distorted when she is in labor. The hot compress should be wrapped in a towel or pad, and before placing it on the woman's skin the temperature of the compress should be tested on the caregiver's own inner forearm.

7

## Hydrotherapy

*Note:* Hydrotherapy (Figs 7.13, 7.14) often results in dramatic pain reduction and may enhance labor progress. See page 170 for instructions on hydrotherapy.

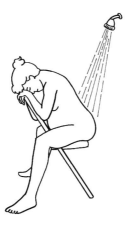

**Fig. 7.13** Shower.

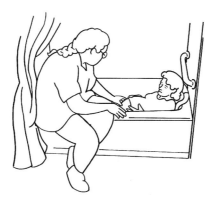

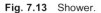

**7**

**Fig. 7.14** Bath.

## Movement

The lunge (Chapter 6, page 154), slow dancing (Chapter 6, page 157), walking (Chapter 6, page 156), pelvic rocking, pelvic tilt (page 152), swaying, rocking (Chapter 6, page 162), the open knee–chest (Chapter 6, page 139), the abdominal lift (Chapter 6, page 160), and abdominal stroking (Chapter 6, page 158) all encourage fetal rotation, and some also relieve back pain. See Figs 7.15–7.17.

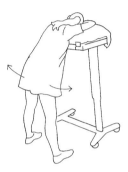

**Fig. 7.15**  Standing, swaying with a tray table.

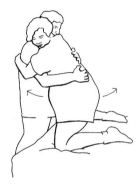

**Fig. 7.16**  Kneeling, rocking with partner support.

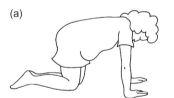

**Fig. 7.17**  Pelvic rocking.

## Birth ball

The birth ball (Figs 7.18–7.19) is an excellent aid to movement and relaxation during labor. It is a physical therapy ball. Unlike large balls made for children's use, physical therapy balls are made to support adult weights. Such balls usually have a 300 lb (136 kg) weight limit,

**7**

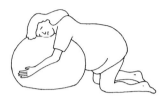

**Fig. 7.18** Kneeling with a ball.

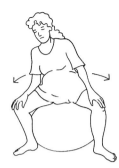

**Fig. 7.19** Sitting swaying on a ball.

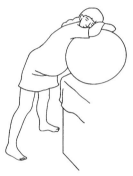

**Fig. 7.20** Standing, leaning on a ball.

but you should check with the seller or manufacturer if the information is not included with the ball. The most widely used size is 65 cm in diameter. For women taller than 5 feet 10 inches (178 cm), a 75 cm diameter is a better choice. Birth balls can be inflated to varying degrees of firmness, according to the woman's comfort.

The round shape of the ball makes swaying (while sitting on it or leaning over it) almost effortless. It is a wonderful alternative to the hands-and-knees position. Cover the ball with a waterproof bed pad, towel or blanket. The ball can be cleaned with the same disinfectant used on the birthing bed mattress.

*Caution:* The first few times a woman sits on the ball, she may feel a bit unsteady. She should hold on to the bed or her partner until she is totally secure. Also, as she sits on the ball, she should hold it to be sure it does not roll away! If insecure while sitting on the ball, she may prefer to use it in a kneeling or standing position, as shown in Figs 7.18 and 7.20. Some childbirth classes provide balls for expectant parents to try before labor.

Some parents buy a ball for their own use in labor and afterwards. The ball is very soothing for a fussy baby, when the parent sits on the ball with the baby nestled into his or her shoulder and bounces gently. It is much easier on the parent's back than walking with the baby.

## Transcutaneous electrical nerve stimulation (TENS)

TENS units (Fig. 7.21) are available from physical therapy clinics and from medical equipment rental companies.

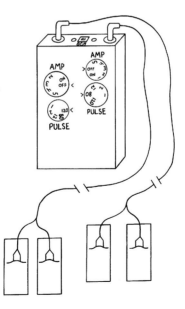

**Fig. 7.21** TENS unit.

***How:*** The four stimulating pads, or electrodes, are placed on the low back on the paraspinal muscles on either side of the spine, two at the level of the lowest ribs and two slightly above the level of the gluteal cleft (Fig. 7.22). The TENS unit has several adjustable parameters: the mode, the width, the frequency, and the intensity. The unit usually comes with instructions on these settings. The woman should have professional guidance from a physical therapist or other knowledgeable professional in using a TENS unit in labor.

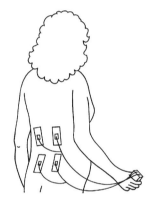

**Fig. 7.22**   TENS in use.

The woman or her partner increases the intensity of the nerve stimulation during contractions, and decreases it between contractions. She feels a 'buzzing,' prickly or tingling sensation, which is kept below painful levels. To avoid habituating to the TENS, the settings (mode, width, and frequency) can be varied to give different sensations.

*Fetal monitoring:* Sometimes the TENS unit interferes with transmission of ultrasound fetal monitor signals. If this is a problem, it can be dealt with by discontinuing the stimulation temporarily so that clear signals are obtained.

### How TENS helps

TENS stimulates tactile nerve endings, and inhibits awareness of pain, according to the Gate Control Theory of Pain[20]. TENS also increases local endorphin production. It appears to have greater benefit if started early in labor.

### When to use TENS

- TENS seems to be more effective when started early, so it makes sense for the woman to obtain her TENS unit and be instructed in its use before labor begins. Then she can begin using it early in labor.
- Throughout labor as long as the woman finds it helpful.

### When not to use TENS

- When using hydrotherapy
- When woman reports that the TENS is not helping. (She may want to turn it off for a while without removing it. She may discover that the contractions are more painful without it.)

### Effectiveness of TENS

Trials of TENS have produced mixed evaluations of benefit[21]. While some trials have found fewer requests for epidural analgesia from TENS users than the comparison groups, other trials found that some women reported greater pain. It appears that TENS is beneficial to some women and not to others. Acceptance of TENS by laboring women and their plans to use it in a future labor appear higher than its overall measurable pain-relieving effect[21,22]. Clearly, further study is needed to determine the most effective way (if any) to use TENS, but in the meantime, women's individual preferences should be respected.

## Intradermal sterile water injections for back pain (I-D water blocks)

Intradermal injections of sterile water are an effective method of reducing back pain[23,24,25] and are easily performed by clinical personnel.

***How***[25]: *Equipment:* alcohol swabs, and a tuberculin syringe with a 25 gauge needle, filled with 0.4 ml of sterile water.

(1) Locate the injection sites (Fig. 7.23). The first two injection sites are located over the posterior superior iliac spines (where the

7

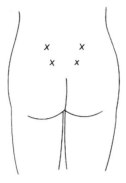

**Fig. 7.23**    Intradermal sterile water injection sites.

'dimples of Venus' are located). The other two sites are located 2 to 3 cm below, and 1 to 2 cm medial to the first two points. A ball point pen can be used to mark each site with an 'X'.

(2)    After swabbing the site with alcohol, a qualified professional injects 0.1 ml of sterile water intradermally (*not* subcutaneously), close to, but not directly on each 'X', to form four small blebs in the skin. The four injections should be performed quickly, to reduce the duration of the pain from the injections.

(3)    The woman will experience intense stinging lasting less than 30 seconds. If the injections are given during a contraction, the stinging is less noticeable. The woman should be told to expect the stinging.

(4)    Within 2 minutes she will experience relief of back pain, lasting 60–90 minutes. The technique can be repeated.

### *How I-D water blocks help*

The mechanism of pain reduction with I-D water blocks is not known. Hypotheses include a rapid increase in local endorphin production, or inhibition of awareness of labor pain (as hypothesized in the gate control theory of pain). However, 90% of women report significant relief of back pain lasting from 45 to 90 minutes after receiving an I-D water block. This technique has also been used to relieve pain from kidney stones[26]

### When to use I-D water blocks

- When woman reports back pain.

### When not to use I-D water blocks

- When woman refuses.

### Effectiveness of intradermal sterile water injections

Effectiveness of I-D water blocks has been demonstrated in two randomized placebo trials[23,24]. Risks of I-D water blocks are the same as with any needle puncture of the skin (minimal when proper technique is used).

## BREATHING FOR RELAXATION AND A SENSE OF MASTERY

### Simple techniques to teach on the spot in labor

Many women have attended childbirth preparation classes, and have already learned some breathing techniques to use in labor. The caregiver should ask them what they learned and encourage the women to use what is already familiar to them. Those women who have not learned any breathing techniques beforehand can be quickly taught some simple effective breathing patterns, and then assisted in using them during contractions.

**How:** We recommend that the caregiver be able to teach two breathing patterns: slow and light.

- *Slow breathing* should be begun at the point in labor when the woman cannot walk or talk through her contractions without pausing over the peaks. Teach her to 'sigh' her way through the contractions with full, easy, audible breaths that may or may not be accompanied by moaning. Combine breathing with imagery: ('Every out breath is a relaxing breath.' 'Send each in-breath to a tense area and breathe the tension away from that area.' 'Imagine that each breath is another step up the mountain, that is, your contraction. When you get to the peak, you can breathe your way

7

down.' 'Let's count your breaths as you go through the contractions. Then (assuming the contractions follow a fairly consistent pattern) we'll be able to tell when you are about halfway through. It will make your contractions seem shorter.').

- *Light breathing* is reserved for a time in active labor when the woman finds that the slow breathing is no longer helping very much, even with your encouragement and help. Teach her to breathe more lightly and more quickly, but still at a speed at which she is comfortable through the contractions. You can pace her with rhythmic hand or head movements, and talk to her soothingly and in the rhythm of her breathing: 'Good, ... that's the way, ... just like that, ... that's right, ... yes....' Hyperventilation is unlikely if you encourage her to keep her inhalations relatively silent and shorter that her exhalations, which should be audible or accompanied by moaning. You can continue the use of guided imagery if she responds well to it.

Of course, you will want her to adapt these rhythmic patterns in whatever way suits her best.

### How breathing techniques help

Breathing in a measured rhythmic pattern is self-calming; it encourages tension release and a sense of well-being. This rhythmic self-calming behavior helps to quieten the cortical activity of the brain, putting the woman in a more instinctual state of mind.

### When to use breathing techniques

- Whenever the woman seems distressed by her contractions
- If she has not mastered any techniques for coping with labor pain.

### When not to use breathing techniques

- If the woman is successfully using other coping techniques or breathing patterns
- If she resists trying them, or cannot respond to your teaching.

# BEARING-DOWN TECHNIQUES FOR THE SECOND STAGE

### *Spontaneous pushing*

Spontaneous pushing is unplanned and unrehearsed by the woman before birth, and undirected during the birth. Her strong involuntary urge to push usually compels her to bear down effectively in synchrony with strong contractions. See Chapter 5 for a full discussion of the rationale for the various approaches to bearing down in the second stage.

*How:* The woman begins breathing in any way that is satisfying to her, and bears down when she has an urge and for as long and as forcefully as her urge demands. Each bearing-down effort usually lasts 5 to 7 seconds. The woman may hold her breath, moan, or bellow during contractions, and may breathe quickly for several seconds between bearing down efforts.

This breathing helps ensure adequate fetal oxygenation. Interestingly, studies have shown it does not lengthen labor significantly, when compared with the prolonged breath-holding and straining that is more the convention today[27].

### *Self-directed pushing*

Sometimes women's spontaneous pushing efforts are ineffective, and self-directed pushing is more productive.

*How:* Self-directed pushing is used when the woman has a spontaneous urge to push but her bearing-down efforts are unfocused, ineffective, and 'diffuse', without apparent progress for 30 minutes. Often her eyes are clenched shut.

First, the caregiver encourages the woman to try a new position. (Gravity-enhancing positions tend to help the woman focus her attention.) If that does not help, the caregiver may instruct the woman to open her eyes and direct her gaze and her efforts toward her vaginal outlet. Without any further direction, the woman frequently responds impressively, becoming much more effective in her bearing-down efforts.

7

### Directed pushing

*How:* With 'directed pushing' the woman is instructed precisely as to when, how, and how long to push. She is usually expected to hold her breath and strain for ten or more seconds at a time with only one short breath between bearing-down efforts. This technique is sometimes referred to as the 'purple pushing,' which describes the color of her face after a few contractions of this type of pushing.

There are potential risks to this type of pushing. See Chapter 5, pages 83–4, for a discussion of these risks. To reduce these risks, the woman should be directed to hold her breath for no more than 5 to 7 seconds at a time, to take several breaths between bearing-down efforts, and to use a position other than lying on her back.

### When to use directed pushing

Directed pushing is used if the woman has no urge to push (as with an epidural), if there is a medical problem requiring that the baby be born right away, or if the woman is unable to focus her efforts to push effectively using self-directed pushing.

## REFERENCES

1. Hodnett, E. (1998) Support from caregivers during childbirth. (Cochrane Review) In: The Cochrane Library (database on disk and CD-ROM), Issue 2. Updated quarterly. The Cochrane Collaboration. Update Software, Oxford.
2. Simkin, P. and Way, K. (1998) DONA Position Paper: The doula's contribution to modern maternity care. Doulas of North America, Seattle.
3. Lehmann, J.F. (1982) *Therapeutic Heat and Cold*, 3rd edition. Williams & Wilkins, Baltimore.
4. Kamis, Y., Shaala, S., Damarawy, H., Romia, A., Toppozada, M. (1983) Effect of heat on uterine contractions during normal labor. *Int. J. Gynaecol. Obstet.* **21**, 491–3.
5. Snyder, G., Group Health Cooperative of Puget Sound Biomedical Services (1998) Personal communication.
6. Katz, V.L., Ryder, R.M., Cefalo, R.C., Carmichael, S.C. and Goolsby, R. (1990) A comparison of bed rest and immersion for treating the edema of pregnancy. *Obstet. Gynecol.* **75(2)**, 147–51.
7. Eriksson, M., Mattsson, L.A. and Ladfors, L. (1997) Early or late bath during the first stage of labour: a randomised study of 200 women. *Midwifery* **13**, 146–8.

**7**

8. Nikodem, V.C. (1998) Immersion in water during pregnancy, labour, and birth. (Cochrane Review). In: The Cochrane Library (database on disk and CD-ROM), Issue 2, Updated quarterly. The Cochrane Collaboration. Update Software, Oxford.

9. Cammu, H., Clasen, K. and Van Wettern, L. (1994) Is having a warm bath during labor useful? *Acta Obstet. Gyn. Scand.* **73**, 468–72.

10. Rush, J., Burlock, S., Lambert, K., Loosley-Millman, M., Hutchison, B. and Enkin, M. (1996) The effects of whirlpool baths in labor: A randomized, controlled trial. *Birth* **23(3)**, 136–43.

11. Enkin, M., Keirse, M.J.N.C., Renfrew, M. and Neilson, J. (1995) Control of pain in labour. In: *A Guide to Effective Care in Labour*, 2nd edition. Oxford University Press, Oxford.

12. Klaus, M.H. and Kennell, J.H. (1997) The doula: an essential ingredient of childbirth rediscovered. *Acta Paediatr.* **86**, 1034–6.

13. Bertsch, T.D., Nagashima-Whalen, L., Dykeman, S., Kennell, J.H. and McGrath, S. (1990) Labor supported by first-time fathers: direct observation with a comparison to experienced doulas. *J. Psychosom. Obstet. Gynecol.* **11**, 251–60.

14. Landry, S.H., McGrath, S.K., Kennell, J.H., Martin, S. and Steelman, L. (1998) The effects of doula support during labor on mother–infant interaction at 2 months. *Pediatr. Res.* **43**, 13A.

15. Wolman, W.L., Chalmers, B., Hofmeyr, J. and Nikodem, V.C. (1993) Postpartum depression and companionship in the clinical birth environment: a randomized controlled study. *Am. J. Obstet. Gynecol.* **168**, 1388–93.

16. Hodnett, E. (1996) Nursing support of the laboring woman. *JOGNN* **25(3)**, 257–64.

17. Radin, T.G., Harmon, J.S. and Hanson, D.A. (1993) Nurses' care during labor: Its effect on the cesarean birth rate of healthy nulliparous women. *Birth* **20(1)**, 14–21.

18. Butler, J., Abrams, B., Parker, J., Roberts, J.M. and Laros, R.K. (1993) Supportive nurse–midwife care is associated with a reduced incidence of cesarean section. *Am. J. Obstet. Gynecol.* **168**, 1407–13.

19. Wuitchik, M., Bakal, D. and Lipshitz, J. (1989) The clinical significance of pain and cognitive activity in latent labor. *Obstet. Gynecol.* **73(1)**, 35–42.

20. Melzack, R.D. (1973) *The Puzzle of Pain.* Basic Books, New York.

21. Carroll, D., Tramer, M., McQuay, H., Nye, B. and Moore, A. (1997) Transcutaneous electrical nerve stimulation in labour: A systematic review. *Br. J. Obstet. Gynaecol.* **104**, 167–75.

22. Wraight, A. (1993) Coping with pain. In: Chamberlain, J.G., Wraight, A. and Steer, P. (eds). *Pain and Its Relief in Childbirth.* Churchill Livingstone, Edinburgh.

23. Ader, L., Hansson, B. and Wallin, G. (1990) Parturition pain treated by intracutaneous injections of sterile water. *Pain* **41**, 133–8.

**7**

24. Trolle, B., Moller, M., Kronborg, H. and Thomsen, S. (1991) The effect of sterile water blocks on low back labor pain. *Am. J. Obstet. Gynecol.* **164 (5, Part 1)**, 1277–81.

25. Reynolds, J.L. (1994) Intracutaneous sterile water for back pain in labor. *Can. Fam. Physician* **40**, 1785–92.

26. Odent, M. (1991) Comments on 'Parturition pain treated by intra-cutaneous injections of sterile water,' by L. Ader, B. Handsson and G. Wallin (*Pain* **41** (1990), 133–8). *Pain* **45**, 220.

27. Roberts, J. and Woolley, D. (1996) A second look at the second stage of labor. *JOGNN* **25(5)**, 415–23.

# Index